Copyright © 2018 by Melanie White

All rights reserved.

Published by Melanie White, www.downsizeme.net.au

Disclaimer:

This recipe book can be used as an adjunct to the Downsize Me Program. For more information, visit www.downsizeme.net.au.

The recipes and information in this book are provided for interest and educational purposes only.

Individual nutritional needs vary considerably and this book is not intended to provide prescriptive medical or dietary advice.

Table of Contents

1. Beverages
AK-47 2
Chai Tea Mix 3
Golden Oatmeal Smoothie 4
Grapefruit Breakfast Margarita 5
Orange AC juice 6
Raspberry Macarina (Rivermouth Cafe) 7
Revitalizer (Moruya Health Cafe) 8

2. Breakfasts
Baked Egg with Pesto Mushroom 10
Breakfast Mug Cake 11
Breakfast Tapas 12
Capsi Egg 13
Chia Pudding 14
Flaxible Smoothie 15
Fruity Chia Pudding 16
Life Saver (Hi-Enz) Muesli 17
Ridiculously Good Pancakes 18
Rocking Breakfast Smoothie 19
Sweet Potato and Orange Pancakes 20
Vegan Sweet Potato Pancakes 21

3. Soups
Carrot and Cauliflower Soup 23
Carrot and Fennel Soup 24
Celery Soup 25
Chicken Kale Soup with Probiotic Sauerkraut 26
Souper Soup 27
Vegetable Soup 28

4. Main Meals
Asian Salad with Salmon 30
Bahmi Goreng 31
Beef Meatballs in Tomato Mushroom Sauce (Red Rose Cafe) 32
Chef's Salad with Fruit 33
Chicken and Black Rice Lunchbox 34
Chicken Fritters (The Muffin Shop) 35
Chicken Stir Fry 36

Chicken with Beetroot, Carrot, Apple and Ginger Salad 37
Chimichurri Steak with Lemon Asparagus and Sweet Potato Chips 38
Indian Chicken 39
Indonesian Beef Stir Fry 40
Mushroom Burgers 41
Nasi Goreng 42
Pizza, low fat Chicken 43
Pizza, Supreme 44
Satisfying Chicken Salad 45
Silverbeet Salad Wraps 46
Soft Lamb Tortillas 47
Spaghetti Squash Bolognaise 48
Spring Tuna Salad 49
Summer Stir Fry 50
Surf and Turf with Spicy Avo Sauce 51
Tasty Beef Burgers 52
Tuna Bolognaise 53

5. Salad and Vegetables
Asparagus with Lemon and Almonds 55
Beetslaw 56
Carrot and Hazelnut Salad 57
Carrot and Kale Salad 58
Coleslaw 59
Cucumber and Fennel Salad 60
Eggplant Parmigiana 61
Eggplant, Tomato and Feta Salad (Grumpy and Sweetheart's) 62
Greek Kale Salad 64
Indian Spinach 65
Roasted Sweet Potato and Fig Salad with Balsamic Glaze 66
Shaved Fennel and Kale Salad 67
Simple Avo and Pea Salad 68
Sweet Potato Chips 69
Tabbouleh 70
Winter Greens Salad 71

6. Sauces and Sides
Chimichurri 73
Gremolata 74

Preserved Lemon Dressing 75
Raspberry Jam 76
Spicy Avocado Sauce 77
Super Pesto 78
Tahini Lemon Dressing 79

7. Snacks

Christmas Balls 81
Curried Cauliflower Bites 82
Dukkah 83
Flax Crackers 84
Fruit Jellies 85
Not Toblerone 86
Power Bites 87
Scrumptious Mushroom Walnut Pate 88
Strawberry Roses 89
Zucchini Avocado Hummus 90

8. Desserts

Blood Orange Jelly 92
Blueberry Sorbet 93
Coconut Ice Cream 94
Fruit Icy Poles 95
Grasshopper Mint Slice 96
Mini Pavlovas 97
Orange Coconut Sorbet 98
Raw Boysenberry Cheesecake 99
Strawberry Cheesecakes 100

9. Basics

Almond Milk 102
Beef bone broth 103
Cauliflower Pizza or Tortilla Wrap 104
Preserved Lemon 105
Sauerkraut 106
Whipped Coconut Cream 107

1 Beverages

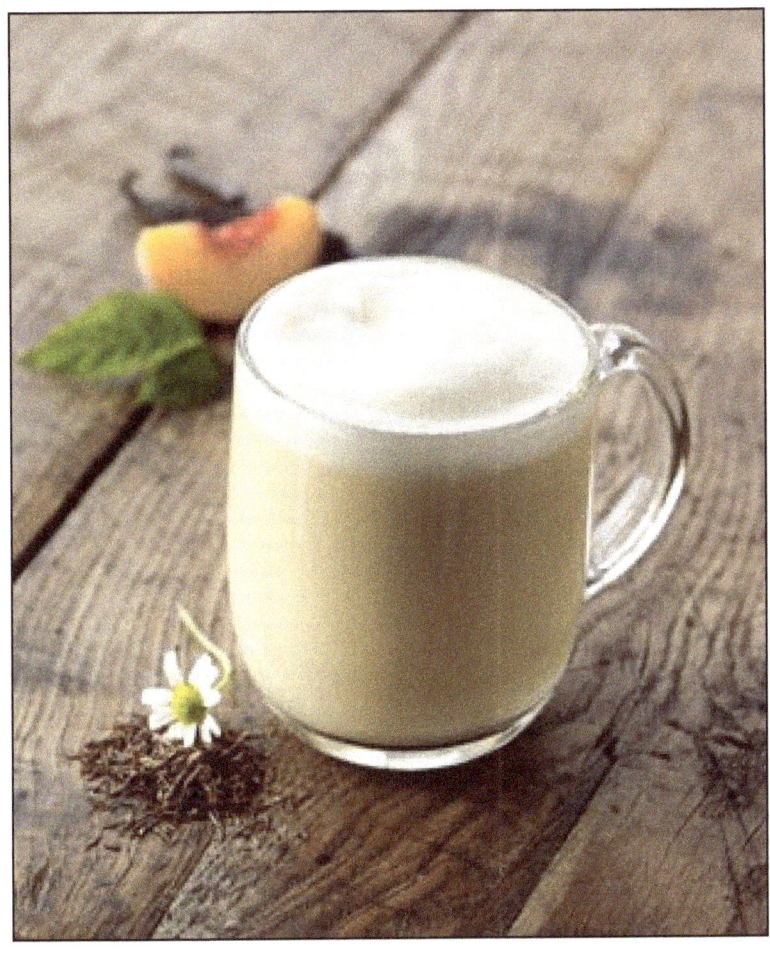

AK-47

1 apple
2 cups kale, torn
1 tsp ginger root

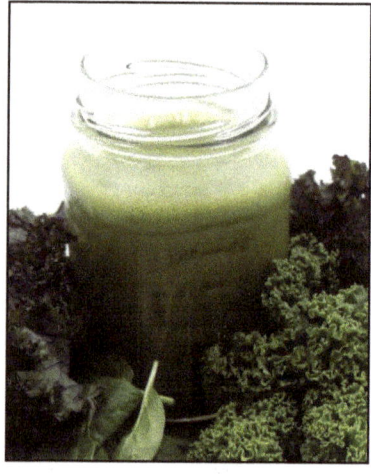

Procedure

1. Juice all ingredients and serve.

Servings: 1

Total Time: 5 minutes

Nutrition Facts

Nutrition (per serving): 106 calories, <1g total fat, 0mg cholesterol, 27.1mg sodium, 484.9mg potassium, 25.3g carbohydrates, 3.4g fibre, 14.4g sugar, 3.3g protein.

DF, GF, V, VG

Recipe Tips

This drink provides a wonderful hit of potassium and vitamin B5.

Chai Tea Mix

3cm ginger root
1/4 tsp peppercorns
1 dried flower star anise
4 cloves
3 cardamom pods
4 pimento seeds
1 vanilla bean pod
1 cinnamon stick
1 tsp licorice root (optional)

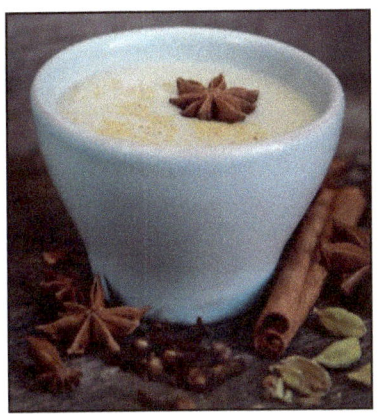

Procedure

1. Blend all ingredients in a coffee/spice grinder to create a thick pulp.
2. Add the pulp to 1.5L water and bring to the boil; simmer 30 minutes.
3. Strain simmered pulp into a glass jar; discard the pulp.
4. The Chai mix can be reheated in a saucepan.
5. Add a black teabag or a rooibos teabag to the hot Chai mix.
6. Serve with honey and almond milk (or hot soy milk), to taste.

Servings: 8

Yield: Enough pulp to make 2L chai tea.

Total Time: 10 minutes

Nutrition Facts

Nutrition (per serving): 16 calories, <1g total fat, 0mg cholesterol, 6.1mg sodium, 66.7mg potassium, 3.7g carbohydrates, 1.8g fibre, <1g sugar, <1g protein.

DF, FOD, GF, V, VG

In Ayurveda, ginger is considered an exceptional digestive aid.

Recipe Tips

If this mix is too spicy, omit the black peppercorns.

Golden Oatmeal Smoothie

100 grams coconut (or Greek) yoghurt

1 cup almond milk

1/2 tsp ground turmeric

1/4 cup rolled oats

1/2 tsp cinnamon

1/2 whole banana

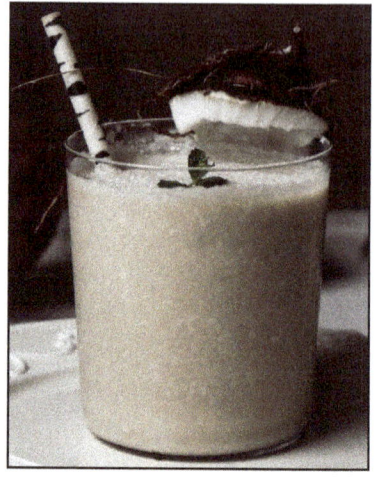

Procedure

1. Blend all ingredients on high speed with a handful of ice until smooth and frothy.
2. Serve immediately.

Total Time: 8 minutes

Nutrition Facts

Nutrition (per serving): 336 calories, 10.8g total fat, 0mg cholesterol, 145.9mg sodium, 456.9mg potassium, 48.8g carbohydrates, 7.6g fibre, 21g sugar, 13.5g protein.

DF, V, VG

Grapefruit Breakfast Margarita

1 grapefruit, juiced
4 ice cubes
100 mL soda water

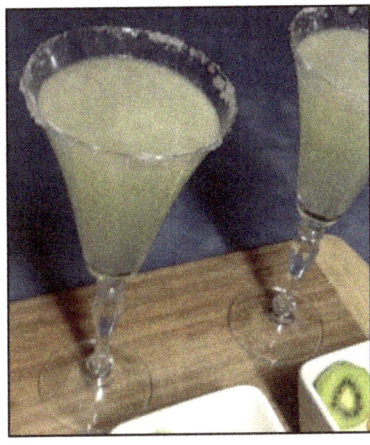

Procedure

1. Blend ingredients.
2. Salt-rim a martini glass and fill with the blended drink.

Servings: 1

Total Time: 5 minutes

Nutrition Facts

Nutrition (per serving): 103 calories, <1g total fat, 0mg cholesterol, 21.4mg sodium, 334.3mg potassium, 26.2g carbohydrates, 3.9g fibre, 17g sugar, 1.9g protein.

DF, FOD, GF, V, VG

A 2014 study shows that grapefruit juice may improve blood glucose and insulin tolerance.
http://www.plosone.org/article/info%3Adoi%2F10.1371%2Fjournal.pone.0108408#s1

Orange AC juice

1 orange, chopped
1 carrot
1/2 lemon

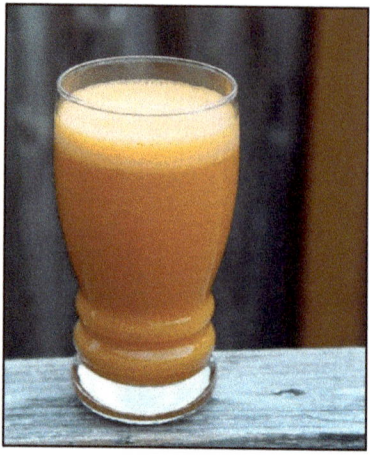

Servings: 1

Total Time: 5 minutes

Nutrition Facts

Nutrition (per serving): 134 calories, <1g total fat, 0mg cholesterol, 59.1mg sodium, 575.4mg potassium, 32.7g carbohydrates, 9.5g fibre, 3.9g sugar, 2.9g protein.

DF, FOD, GF, V, VG

One fresh orange contains 93% of your daily recommended intake of vitamin C (www.whfoods.com).

Raspberry Macarina (Rivermouth Cafe)

1/2 cup raspberries, frozen
1 tsp coconut flakes
1 banana
1 tsp chia seeds
1 tsp L.S.A
1 tsp almond meal
1 tsp Maca powder
1 pinch cinnamon
1/2 tsp honey (optional)
250 ml almond milk

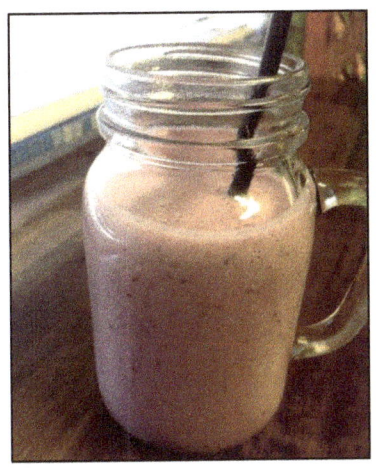

Procedure

1. Blend all ingredients except milk, then add milk at the end and enjoy!

Servings: 1

Total Time: 5 minutes

Nutrition Facts

Nutrition (per serving): 342 calories, 15.8g total fat, 0mg cholesterol, 107.4mg sodium, 752mg potassium, 48.5g carbohydrates, 13.2g fibre, 29.6g sugar, 7.6g protein.

DF, FOD, GF, V, VG

Rheosmin in raspberries may increase metabolism in fat cells and may reduce the risk of obesity and fatty liver (www.whfoods.com).

* Low FODMAP recipe if honey is omitted

Recipe Tips

Add ice for a frosty cold smoothie.

Source

Source: Thanks to Tina McDonald at the Rivermouth Cafe, Tomakin, for donating this recipe.
http://www.therivermouthstore.com.au/

Revitalizer (Moruya Health Cafe)

1 small beetroot

1 small apple, green, cored and chopped

1 small carrot

5 medium celery stalks

1 ginger root, 1cm slice (optional)

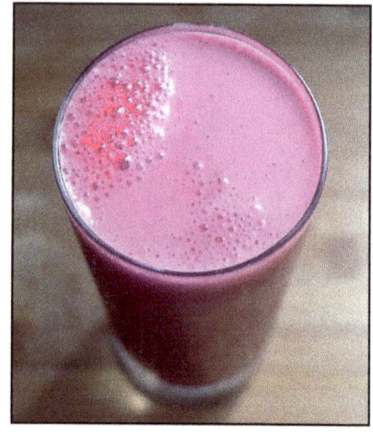

Procedure

1 Juice with ice until smooth - enjoy!

Servings: 1

Total Time: 5 minutes

Nutrition Facts

Nutrition (per serving): 148 calories, <1g total fat, 0mg cholesterol, 279.8mg sodium, 1133.2mg potassium, 34.3g carbohydrates, 9.9g fibre, 23.1g sugar, 3.7g protein.

DF, GF, V, VG

Beetroots are a unique source of betalains, which provide antioxidant, anti-inflammatory and detoxification support (www.whfoods.com).

Source

Source: Thanks to Gemma Cassidy at Moruya Health Cafe for donating this recipe. https://www.facebook.com/pages/Moruya-Health-Cafe/194192833972805

2 Breakfasts

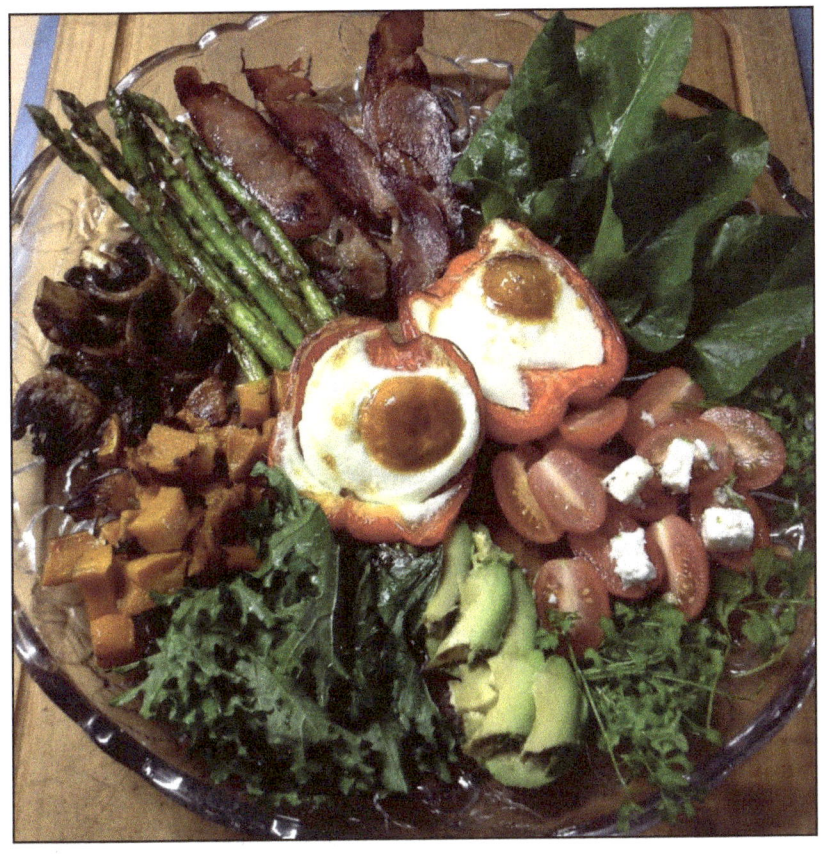

Baked Egg with Pesto Mushroom

1 mushroom, field, whole
1 tbsp super pesto
1 egg
1 tbsp Goat's feta, crumbled

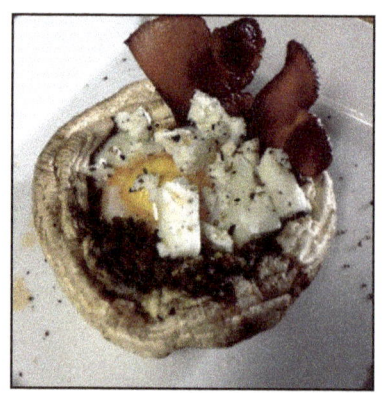

Procedure

1. Preheat the oven to 180 degrees Celsius.
2. Wipe the mushroom to remove any soil and remove the stem.
3. Place the mushroom on a non-stick tray.
4. Smear the inner edge of the mushroom with pesto.
5. Crack the egg into the centre of the mushroom.
6. Place the mushroom into the oven and bake for 15 minutes, until the egg is cooked, and the mushroom is tender.
7. Crumble goat's feta over the top and serve. Crispy lean bacon makes a nice garnish.

Servings: 1

Total Time: 20 minutes

Nutrition Facts

Nutrition (per serving): 175 calories, 13.1g total fat, 193.9mg cholesterol, 244.5mg sodium, 279.6mg potassium, 4.1g carbohydrates, 2.9g fibre, 1.2g sugar, 10.2g protein.

GF, V

Eggs are a nutrient-rich, whole food that contains protein of high biological value, fat, vitamin D and omega 3 fatty acids. Free range, organic eggs are best.

Breakfast Mug Cake

1 tbsp almond meal

1 tbsp cacao powder (rounded spoons)

1 whole egg

1/2 banana

1/2 tsp vanilla extract

1 tbsp milk

2 tbsp blueberries (optional)

1 tsp coconut flakes (optional)

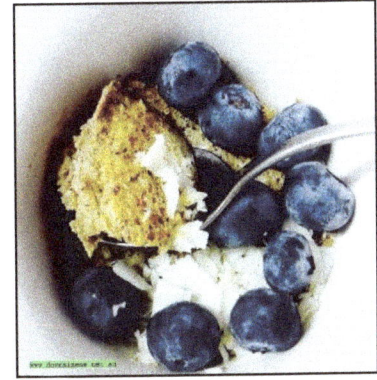

Procedure

1. Mash the banana until pulpy.
2. Combine banana and all other ingredients except berries and coconut: mix thoroughly until smooth and well combined.
3. Microwave for one minute.
4. Top with blueberries and coconut - enjoy warm.

Servings: 1

Yield: 1 cup

Total Time: 4 minutes

Nutrition Facts

Nutrition (per serving): 271 calories, 15.2g total fat, 187.2mg cholesterol, 83.9mg sodium, 432.3mg potassium, 25.1g carbohydrates, 6.1g fibre, 13.5g sugar, 10.8g protein.

Breakfast Tapas

2 serves Capsi Egg

2 rashers short cut bacon rasher

2 serves Asparagus with Lemon and Almonds

3/4 cup mushrooms, sliced

1 cup kale leaves, torn

1 cup silverbeet (chard), raw

1/2 cup watercress leaves

10 cherry tomatoes, halved

1/2 avocado, sliced

2/3 cup sweet potato, cubed, baked

1 tbsp lemon juice

Tabasco sauce to taste

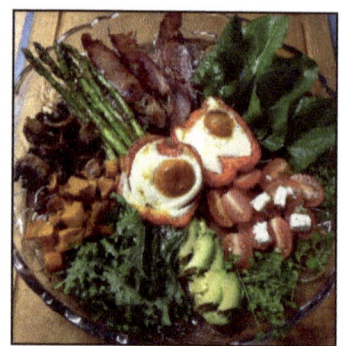

Procedure

1. Preheat the griller and place a non-stick pan over medium heat.
2. Crisp extra-lean bacon in the pan.
3. Place capsicum cut-side down on a tray and grill under medium heat to blacken skin, remove then turn capsicum over and crack egg into the shell.
4. Place capsicum under the grill; check regularly as you proceed.
5. Meanwhile, fry mushroom and asparagus for 5 - 7 minutes, then grate lemon zest over asparagus.
6. Slice and arrange cherry tomatoes on platter with avocado and cress.
7. Turn the mushrooms, asparagus and bacon; cook 5 minutes.
8. Add sweet potato, kale and silverbeet to pan to wilt (5 - 7 mins).
9. Arrange the vegetables on the platter, add bacon and capsi-eggs. Serve with Tabasco sauce and pesto (optional).

Servings: 2

Total Time: 25 minutes

Nutrition Facts

Nutrition (per serving): 405 calories, 19.9g total fat, 186mg cholesterol, 540.4mg sodium, 2044.9mg potassium, 43.7g carbohydrates, 12.6g fibre, 10.4g sugar, 20.7g protein.

DF, GF

Capsi Egg

1 half red capsicum

1 whole egg

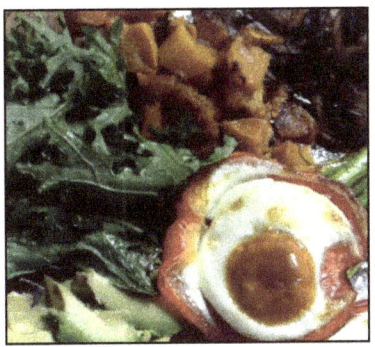

Procedure

1. Turn the grill on to medium.
2. Place the capsicum half, cut side down, on a small baking tray.
3. Grill for 5 minutes until the skin starts to blister; blanch in cold water and peel.
4. Put piece of baking paper on the tray.
5. Put the capsicum, cut side up, on the tray.
6. Crack the egg into the capsicum cup and grill for 5 - 10 minutes to desired firmness.

Servings: 1

Total Time: 15 minutes

Nutrition Facts

Nutrition (per serving): 94 calories, 5g total fat, 186mg cholesterol, 73.9mg sodium, 222.1mg potassium, 4.7g carbohydrates, 1.5g fibre, 3.2g sugar, 7g protein.

DF, FOD, GF, V

Recipe Tips

This could be prepared with 2 egg whites instead of a whole egg. Delicious served with grilled mushrooms and Super Pesto.

Chia Pudding

2 tbsp chia seeds
100 mL coconut milk, light
100 grams blueberries
1 tsp cacao nibs
1 pinch stevia (optional)

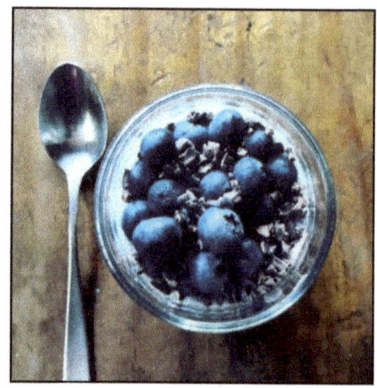

Procedure

1. Mix chia seeds and coconut milk (and stevia if using).
2. Refrigerate 5 – 10 minutes.
3. Serve with fresh berries and cacao nibs.

Servings: 1

Total Time: 10 minutes

Nutrition Facts

Nutrition (per serving): 354 calories, 24.4g total fat, 0mg cholesterol, 5.5mg sodium, 227.4mg potassium, 31.2g carbohydrates, 13.7g fibre, 11.7g sugar, 7.7g protein.

DF, FOD, GF, V, VG

Chia seeds are good source of omega-3 fats and fibre and contain a modest amount of protein. These seeds contain 21 of the 22 amino acids (www.nutritiondata.self.com).

Flaxible Smoothie

1/2 banana
1/2 cup strawberries
1 tbsp cacao powder
1 avocado, peeled
1 cup spinach leaves
2 tsp flax seeds
1 cup almond milk

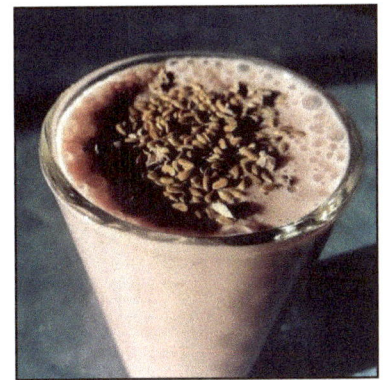

Servings: 1

Total Time: 5 minutes

Nutrition Facts

Nutrition (per serving): 485 calories, 36.1g total fat, 0mg cholesterol, 141.4mg sodium, 1555.4mg potassium, 40.7g carbohydrates, 20.8g fibre, 19.5g sugar, 9.5g protein.

Fruity Chia Pudding

1 tbsp chia seeds

100 mL orange juice, freshly squeezed

100 grams mixed berries

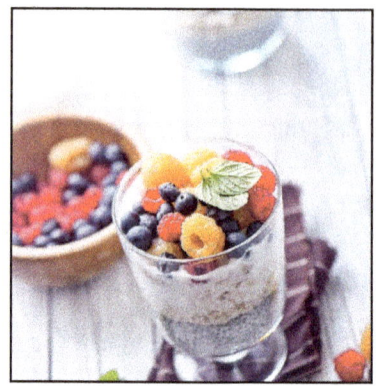

Procedure

1. Mix chia seeds and orange juice.
2. Refrigerate for at least 30 minutes; serve with fresh berries.

Servings: 1

Total Time: 35 minutes

Nutrition Facts

Nutrition (per serving): 151 calories, 3.6g total fat, 0mg cholesterol, 3.6mg sodium, 317.7mg potassium, 29.1g carbohydrates, 6g fibre, 18.4g sugar, 3.1g protein.

Recipe Tips

* Recipe is low FODMAP if orange juice is <100mL

Life Saver (Hi-Enz) Muesli

1/2 cup quinoa puffs or flakes

1/2 cup amaranth puffs or flakes

1/2 cup buckwheat, roasted

1/2 cup coconut flakes

1/4 cup sunflower seeds, raw

1/4 cup pepitas, roughly chopped

1/4 cup chia seeds

1/2 cup almonds, raw, chopped

1/2 cup cashews, raw, chopped

1/2 cup walnuts, raw, chopped

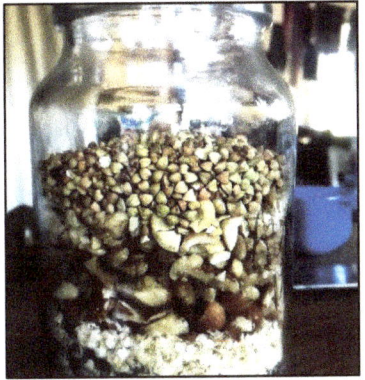

Procedure

1. Mix all ingredients and store in an airtight container.
2. Ideally, soak the next day's serve of cereal overnight in filtered water to activate the nuts and seeds, then drain and serve with almond milk and fresh berries.
3. Alternatively, mix ingredients then toast lightly in a non-stick pan for 5 - 10 minutes, until golden; allow to cool and then store; serve dry with milk and fresh berries.

Servings: 8

Yield: 1/2 cup per serve

Total Time: 45 minutes

Nutrition Facts

Nutrition (per serving): 305 calories, 22.4g total fat, 0mg cholesterol, 7mg sodium, 330.2mg potassium, 21g carbohydrates, 6g fibre, 1.8g sugar, 9.7g protein.

Activating nuts and seeds by soaking them overnight releases enzymes that aid digestion and reduces the phytic acid in the nuts and seeds to make nutrients more available to the body.

Recipe Tips

Replace cashews with peanuts for a different flavour.

Ridiculously Good Pancakes

3 tbsp whole meal spelt flour

1 whole egg

4 tbsp Greek yoghurt

1 pinch baking soda (bicarb soda)

1 spray coconut oil spray

3/4 cup blueberries

1 tsp cacao nibs

1 tbsp maple syrup

1 tbsp coconut flakes (sulphur-free)

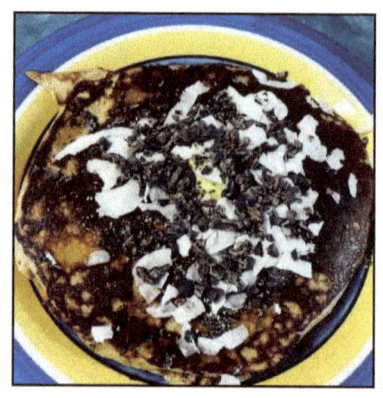

Procedure

1. Mix flour, yoghurt, egg and baking powder well with a whisk to get a thick consistency.
2. Leave the mixture to sit for 5 minutes until bubbles start to form.
3. Spray a non-stick pan with coconut or olive oil and heat to medium.
4. Pour in half the mix and leave to sit until bubbles start to form; flip and cook the other side.
5. Plate the first pancake and cover with foil. Repeat cooking process with the other half of the mixture.
6. Plate the second pancake on top of the first.
7. Scatter with cacao nibs, coconut flakes, maple syrup and blueberries.
8. Serve immediately.

Total Time: 15 minutes

Nutrition Facts

Nutrition (per serving): 431 calories, 16.9g total fat, 186mg cholesterol, 277.6mg sodium, 404mg potassium, 59.2g carbohydrates, 10.8g fibre, 31.8g sugar, 15.7g protein.

Rocking Breakfast Smoothie

50 mL coconut milk
50 grams Greek yoghurt
125 mL water
30 grams protein powder
1 tsp maca powder
4 ice cubes
3/4 cup rock melon

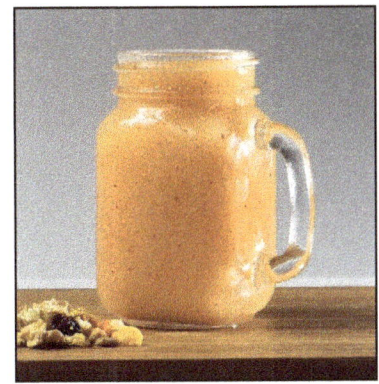

Procedure

1. Blend and serve!

Servings: 1

Total Time: 5 minutes

Nutrition Facts

Nutrition (per serving): 268 calories, 10.3g total fat, 0mg cholesterol, 347.8mg sodium, 446.1mg potassium, 20.5g carbohydrates, 3.1g fibre, 15.2g sugar, 29g protein.

GF, V

Rock melon (also called cantaloupe melon) is a rich source of vitamin A. It may lower the risk of metabolic syndrome (www.whfoods.com).

Sweet Potato and Orange Pancakes

50 grams sweet potato, cooked

1 small orange, peeled, and seeds removed

1 tsp flax seeds, ground

1 tbsp almond meal

1 whole egg

1/2 tsp baking soda

1/2 tsp cinnamon

1/2 tsp vanilla extract

1/2 tsp coconut oil

1 serve Raspberry Jam (topping) (see recipe)

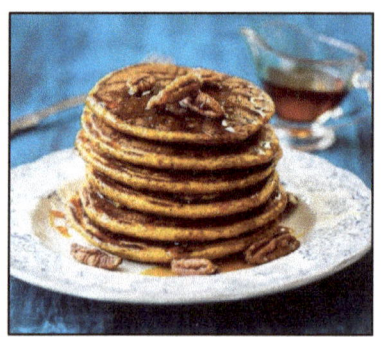

Procedure

1. Blend all ingredients in a food processor or with a stick mixer.
2. Heat coconut oil over medium heat in a non-stick pan.
3. Spoon the pancake mix into the pan (about 3 small pancakes).
4. Cook for 5 minutes before carefully flipping (mixture will be soft).
5. After flipping, place a lid over the fry pan to steam the pancakes.
6. Cook a further 3 - 5 minutes.
7. Serve with Raspberry Jam (optional).

Servings: 1

Total Time: 15 minutes

Nutrition Facts

Nutrition (per serving): 265 calories, 11.7g total fat, 186mg cholesterol, 734.9mg sodium, 565.2mg potassium, 31g carbohydrates, 8.5g fibre, 13.6g sugar, 10.4g protein.

DF, FOD, GF, V

* Recipe is low FODMAP if almond quantity is 1 tablespoon or less This recipe is an excellent source of vitamin A (both retinoids and carotenoids) according to criteria in www.whfoods.org.

Flax seeds are an excellent source of omega 3 fats (alpha-linoleic acid) and a very good source of fibre.

Vegan Sweet Potato Pancakes

1 tbsp flax seeds, ground
1 tbsp chia seeds
3 tbsp boiling water
1/2 tsp cinnamon
1 medium sweet potato, cooked and cooled
1/2 cup blueberries
1 tsp pumpkin seeds

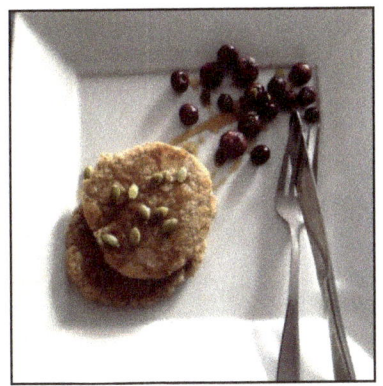

Procedure

1. Mix flax seeds and chia seeds in boiling water; allow to sit 5 minutes.
2. Heat a non-stick fry pan or barbecue grill to medium, add coconut oil.
3. Blend seeds with sweet potato until smooth.
4. Divide the mix into two portions and smear over the grill/pan, smoothing into 1cm thick circles with the back of a desert spoon.
5. Cook 2 - 3 minutes, then flip.
6. Cook the other side for 2 - 3 minutes.
7. Serve with blueberries, pumpkin seeds and maple syrup if desired.

Servings: 2

Yield: 2 pancakes

Total Time: 15 minutes

Nutrition Facts

Nutrition (per serving): 136 calories, 3.7g total fat, 0mg cholesterol, 187.7mg sodium, 450.9mg potassium, 23.6g carbohydrates, 5.8g fibre, 12.1g sugar, 3.5g protein.

DF, FOD, GF, V, VG

Flax can be used as an egg substitute; mix 1 tbsp flax with 3 tbsp water, whisk and leave to stand 2 – 3 minutes before using.

3 Soups

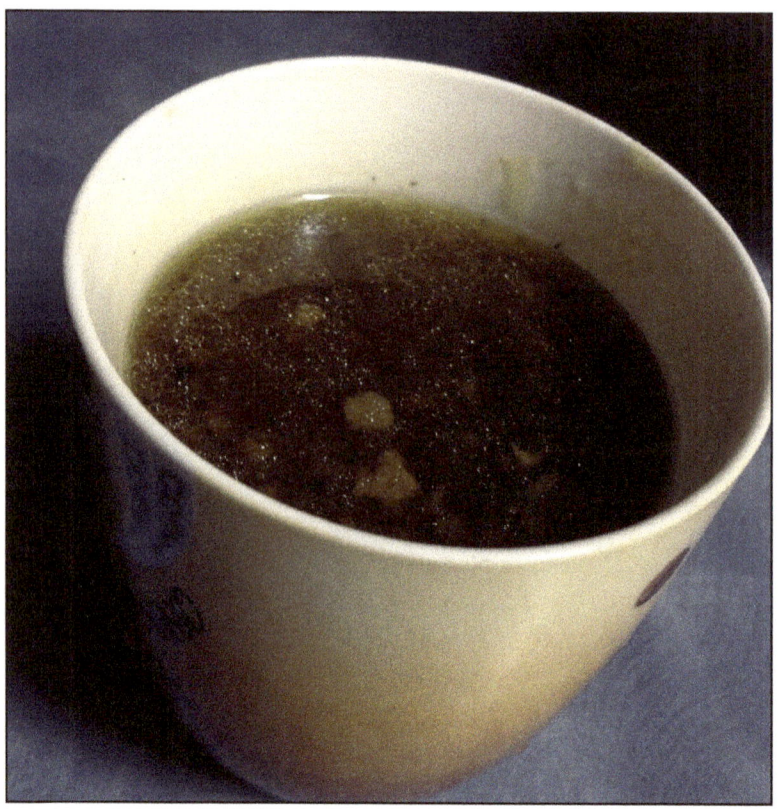

Carrot and Cauliflower Soup

3 carrots, cut into pieces
1/2 cauliflower
1 cup water
1/2 cup bone broth (or stock)
100 mL coconut milk, light
1 garlic clove, crushed
2 spring onions, finely chopped
1 sprig coriander
1/2 tsp cumin seeds

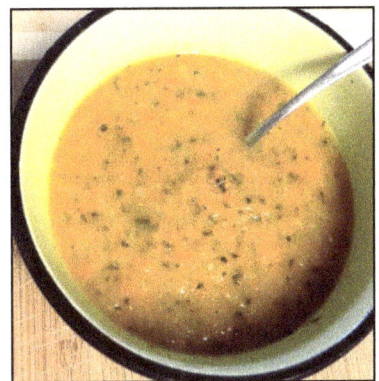

Procedure

1. Dry fry garlic in a pan with spring onions.
2. Add chopped carrot and cauliflower and sauté until browned.
3. Transfer garlic, onions, carrot and cauliflower to a pot.
4. Add remaining ingredients except cumin; simmer gently for 5 minutes.
5. Blend soup; dish into bowls and top with a sprinkle of cumin.

Servings: 2

Total Time: 25 minutes

Nutrition Facts

Nutrition (per serving): 235 calories, 8.7g total fat, 2mg cholesterol, 218.7mg sodium, 1619mg potassium, 35g carbohydrates, 11.8g fibre, 14.8g sugar, 10.4g protein.

DF, GF

Recipe Tips

Convert to a vegan or vegetarian recipe by replacing bone broth with homemade vegetable stock.

Carrot and Fennel Soup

2 carrots, chopped

1/2 fennel bulbs, chopped

4 kale leaves, de-stemmed and torn

1 cup bone broth

1 pinch Himalayan salt

1 tsp cumin seeds

100 grams chicken breast, cooked, diced

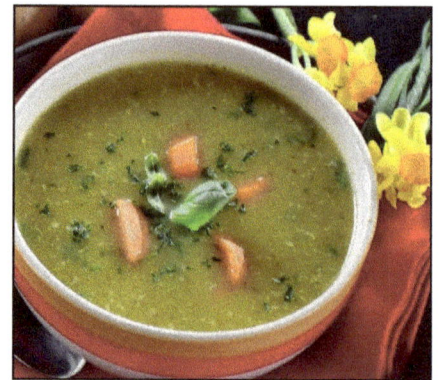

Procedure

1. Cook all ingredients except chicken cumin seed in a saucepan for 10 minutes.
2. Puree with a stick mixer or food processor.
3. Add cooked chicken cubes and cook 5 minutes.
4. Transfer to a bowl and top with cumin seeds.

Servings: 1

Total Time: 20 minutes

Nutrition Facts

Nutrition (per serving): 316 calories, 6.2g total fat, 72mg cholesterol, 673.5mg sodium, 1973.9mg potassium, 37g carbohydrates, 10.2g fibre, 10.8g sugar, 31g protein.

DF, FOD, GF

Cumin seeds are an excellent source of iron and may benefit the digestive system. They are used in Ayurvedic medicine for to reduce gas and bloating (Dr. David Frawley, 2014).

Celery Soup

6 stalks celery, leaves included
1/2 onion
1/2 bulb fennel (small bulb)
1 sprig coriander leaves
4 tbsp coconut milk
1 cup chicken stock, home made
1/2 tsp coconut oil

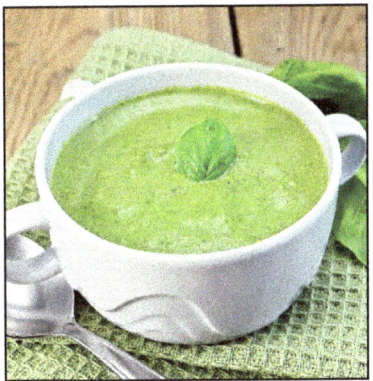

Procedure

1. Heat coconut oil in a saucepan over medium heat.
2. Stir-fry onion until translucent.
3. Transfer onions to a food processor with all other ingredients - pulse until smooth and creamy.
4. Transfer mixture back to the saucepan and simmer for 10 minutes.
5. Garnish with coriander or basil leaves.

Servings: 2

Total Time: 20 minutes

Nutrition Facts

Nutrition (per serving): 166 calories, 9.2g total fat, 3.6mg cholesterol, 315.8mg sodium, 843.8mg potassium, 17.1g carbohydrates, 4.6g fibre, 5.7g sugar, 5.5g protein.

DF, GF

Celery is a good source of specific phytonutrients which are known to reduce oxidative damage and inflammatory reactions in the digestive tract (www.whfoods.com).

Recipe Tips

Convert to a vegan/vegetarian recipe by using vegetable stock.

Chicken Kale Soup with Probiotic Sauerkraut

100 grams chicken breast, diced

1 whole leek, white only, chopped

1 garlic clove, crushed

1 cup kale, torn

1 cup green beans, trimmed and cut in half

1 tsp wholegrain mustard

1 tsp lemon juice

1 small chili pepper, finely chopped

1 tbsp apple cider vinegar

2 cups water

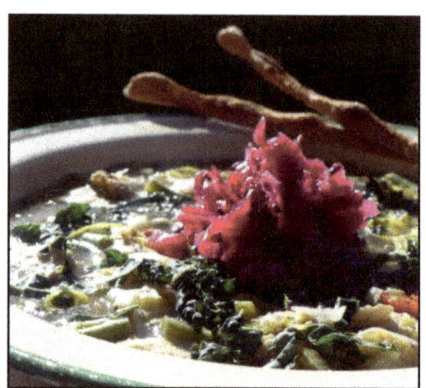

Procedure

1. Cook the chicken breast cubes in a large pot over medium heat until cooked through. Use a little bit of water to avoid sticking.
2. Add leek and garlic to the pot and stir well to brown.
3. Add kale, beans, mustard, lemon, chilli and stir quickly for one minute.
4. Add vinegar and water; simmer the soup for 15 minutes.
5. Serve with sauerkraut and grissini sticks.

Total Time: 45 minutes

Nutrition Facts

Nutrition (per serving): 267 calories, 4.4g total fat, 64mg cholesterol, 253.5mg sodium, 1275.8mg potassium, 31.9g carbohydrates, 5.4g fibre, 9.7g sugar, 28.9g protein.

DF, GF

Kale is a cruciferous vegetable (e.g. broccoli family). It is a rich source of many vitamins and minerals, and is known for its ability to lower cholesterol, reduce cancer risk and support detoxification.

Souper Soup

1 serve Bone broth
1 garlic clove, crushed
1 onion, finely diced
125 grams sweet potato, cubed
1 cup kale stalks, finely diced
1 bay leaf
1 tsp tarragon leaves

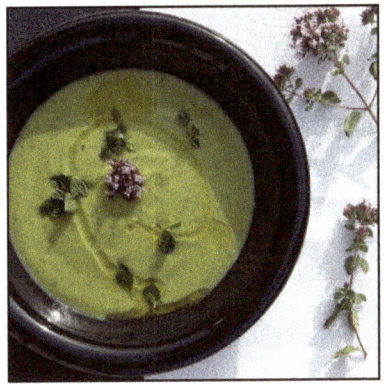

Procedure

1. Dry-fry garlic and onion in a non-stick pot.
2. Add sweet potato, kale stalks and bone broth; cook 20 minutes.
3. Add bay leaf and tarragon in the last five minutes of cooking.
4. Remove from heat, blend with a stick mixer.
5. Season to taste before serving.

Servings: 1

Total Time: 35 minutes

Nutrition Facts

Nutrition (per serving): 253 calories, 2.8g total fat, 8mg cholesterol, 165.1mg sodium, 1181mg potassium, 49.8g carbohydrates, 7.7g fibre, 13.5g sugar, 10g protein.

DF, GF

This is a great way of using the nutritious kale stems which are otherwise tough to eat.

Vegetable Soup

1/2 small onion, finely chopped
1/2 tsp olive oil
2 stalks celery, finely chopped
1/2 cup mushrooms, sliced
2 whole carrots, diced
1 small zucchini, cubed
1 cup pumpkin, cubed
1 tsp mixed herbs
1 pinch Himalayan salt
1 cup vegetable stock or bone broth
1 pinch cracked black pepper
3 cups water

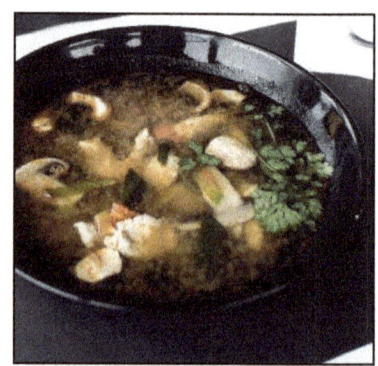

Procedure

1. Heat a heavy-base saucepan over medium heat.
2. Add the diced onion and olive oil and fry until the onion is translucent.
3. Add remaining ingredients to the saucepan; bring to the boil and then reduce heat to a simmer and cook for 20 minutes.
4. Serve immediately - either as is, or blend with a stick mixer if you prefer. Adjust seasoning and top with parsley.

Servings: 1

Total Time: 35 minutes

Nutrition Facts

Nutrition (per serving): 266 calories, 6.4g total fat, 7.2mg cholesterol, 582.9mg sodium, 1938.8mg potassium, 43.7g carbohydrates, 9.3g fibre, 21.7g sugar, 12.8g protein.

4 Main Meals

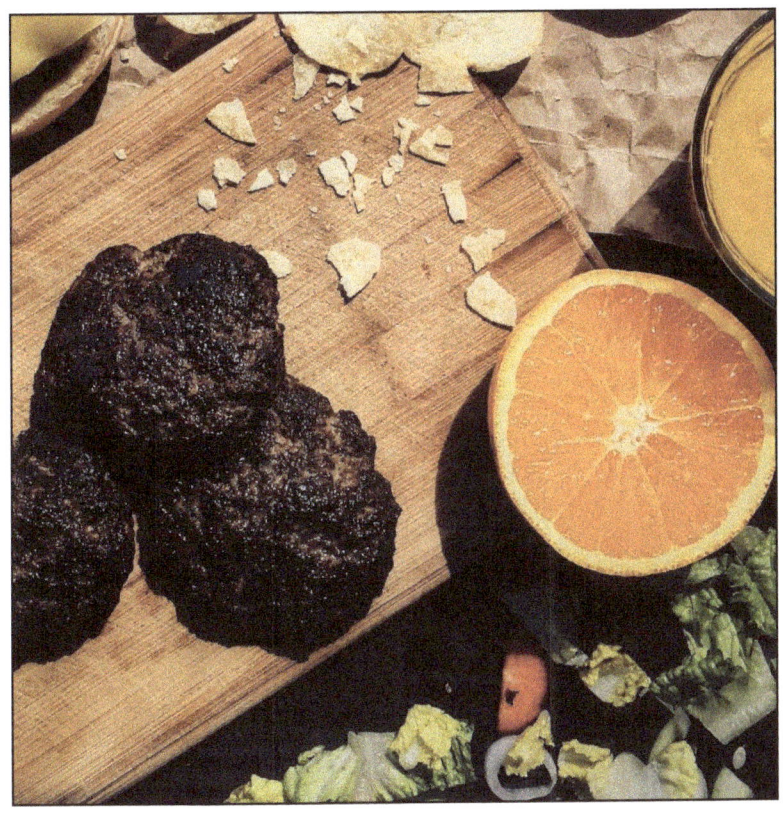

Asian Salad with Salmon

100 grams salmon, hot smoked (or fresh, or canned)

3 cups lettuce, mixed, shredded

5 snow peas, sliced

1 tomato, cut into cubes

1 Lebanese cucumber, diced

2 tsp sesame seeds (dressing)

75 mL rice wine vinegar (dressing)

2 tbsp lemon juice (dressing)

2 tsp ginger, grated (dressing)

1 pinch stevia (optional)

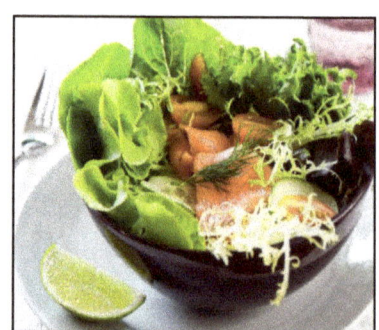

Procedure

1. Prepare lettuce, snow peas, tomato and cucumber, top with salmon.
2. Mix dressing ingredients and pour over the top, server immediately.

Servings: 1

Total Time: 10 minutes

Nutrition Facts

Nutrition (per serving): 262 calories, 8.6g total fat, 23mg cholesterol, 2028.8mg sodium, 1963.5mg potassium, 53.2g carbohydrates, 6.9g fibre, 10.9g sugar, 25.3g protein.

DF, GF

Salmon is an excellent source of protein and omega 3 fatty acids.

Source

Thanks to Jane Allen of The Muffin Shop for donating this recipe.

www.themuffinshop.com.au

Bahmi Goreng

2 serves Slim Pasta
1 egg white, lightly beaten
1/4 cup soy sauce or Bragg's
2 garlic cloves, crushed
4 shallots, coarsely chopped
50 grams chicken breast, sliced
100 grams pork fillet
10 anchovy fillets, dried
80 grams cabbage, shredded
½ carrot, shredded
2 chili, red, chopped
60 ml vegetable stock
1/2 cup bean sprouts

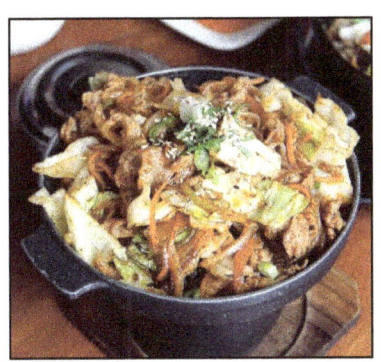

Procedure

1. Drain Slim Pasta and cover with boiling water; set aside.
2. Heat a non-stick pan to medium.
3. Mix beaten egg with 1 tbsp of the soy sauce and cook omelette; remove from pan, roll up, slice thinly.
4. Stir-fry garlic cloves and spring onions until tender; remove from pan.
5. Add chicken thighs and pork fillet; brown and cook through.
6. Add cabbage, carrot, chilli and stir-fry until just cooked.
7. Add stock and remaining soy sauce, stir through.
8. Drain Slendier Pasta, add to the pan, stir well and heat through.
9. Divide mixture between two bowls, top with garlic shallots, dried anchovy, bean sprouts and sliced omelette.
10. Serve with a wedge of lime, fresh chilli and fresh coriander if desired.

Servings: 2

Total Time: 45 minutes

Nutrition Facts

Nutrition (per serving): 721 calories, 3.2g total fat, 51.5mg cholesterol, 1135.4mg sodium, 3330.4mg potassium, 143.1g carbohydrates, 29.4g fibre, 67.1g sugar, 42.2g protein.

DF, GF

Beef Meatballs in Tomato Mushroom Sauce (Red Rose Cafe)

1/2 tsp coconut oil
1/2 garlic clove, crushed
1/2 onion, finely diced
1 can tomatoes (low salt), diced
1 cup mushrooms, sliced
1/2 tsp rosemary, fresh, chopped
1/4 tsp oregano leaves, chopped
1/2 tsp basil leaves, chopped
1/2 tsp cumin seeds, ground
110 grams beef mince, extra lean (Heart Smart) (meatballs)
2 grissini sticks, crushed (meatballs)
1/2 egg white (meatballs)
1/4 cup parsley, chopped (meatballs)
1 pinch each Himalayan salt & pepper (meatballs)
1/2 tsp cumin, ground (meatballs)

Procedure

1. Heat oil; cook garlic & onion on medium heat until transparent.
2. Add tomatoes, herbs, spices, mushrooms and half a cup of water, cook on low heat 20 - 25 minutes until thickened.
3. Once the sauce is cooking, mix meatball ingredients with clean hands and roll into eight evenly-sized balls.
4. Place balls in the sauce and simmer slowly for 20 minutes.
5. Serve with steamed green vegetables or a portion of Slendier pasta, topped with fresh basil and lemon zest.

Servings: 1

Total Time: 45 minutes

Nutrition Facts

Nutrition (per serving): 317 calories, 10.1g total fat, 68.2mg cholesterol, 220.3mg sodium, 1388.9mg potassium, 25.9g carbohydrates, 5.6g fibre, 9.7g sugar, 32.9g protein.

Fresh herbs contain important antioxidants for heart health.

Source

Thanks to Barbara McLean (Red Rose Cafe) for this recipe.

Chef's Salad with Fruit

150 grams chicken thigh, grilled or baked, cut into strips

6 whole cherry tomatoes, halved

2 cups romaine lettuce, roughly chopped

6 whole olives

6 asparagus spears

3 sweet potato slices, cooked, 1cm thick

1 tsp olive oil

1 tbsp white wine vinegar

1/2 cup cherries, pitted, halved

1/2 mango, peeled, seeded and chopped

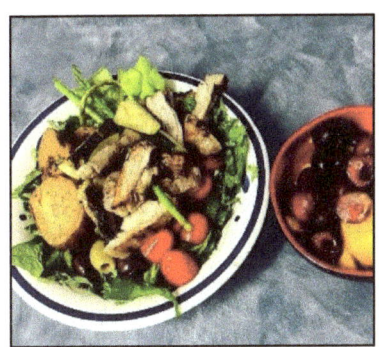

Procedure

1. Arrange the lettuce, tomato, olives, asparagus and sweet potato in a bowl.
2. Top with cooked chicken slices (or cook then slice).
3. Combine the oil and white wine vinegar and drizzle over the top.
4. Combine the mango and cherries in a separate bowl.
5. Serve immediately.

Servings: 1

Total Time: 25 minutes (includes time to cook chicken)

Nutrition Facts

Nutrition (per serving): 464 calories, 14.6g total fat, 142.5mg cholesterol, 416.3mg sodium, 1598.5mg potassium, 52.6g carbohydrates, 11g fibre, 31.1g sugar, 35.6g protein.

Chicken and Black Rice Lunchbox

150 grams chicken thigh, grilled or baked and sliced

1/4 avocado, diced

1 cup mixed lettuce leaves

1/2 cup black rice, cooked according to directions

pinch salt and pepper to taste

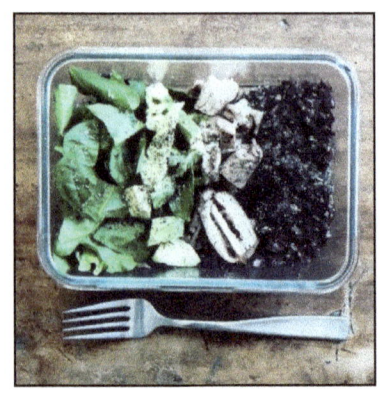

Procedure

1. Chop all ingredients and arrange in a lunch box.
2. Refrigerate until ready for use.

Servings: 1

Total Time: 5 minutes

Nutrition Facts

Nutrition (per serving): 417 calories, 14.4g total fat, 142.5mg cholesterol, 432.7mg sodium, 675.3mg potassium, 38.9g carbohydrates, 5.7g fibre, 1.1g sugar, 35.3g protein.

Chicken Fritters (The Muffin Shop)

500 grams chicken breast, minced

1 bunch coriander

1/4 capsicum, red

1/2 Spanish onion

1 tbsp lemon juice

1 tsp ginger, minced

1 pinch chilli flakes

1 egg

2 scoops whey protein isolate powder

1 tsp coconut oil

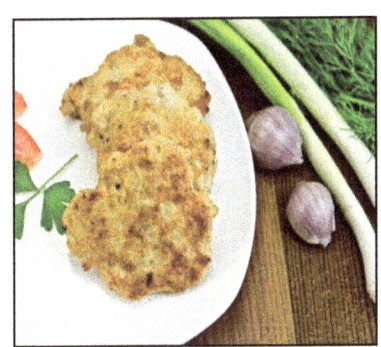

Procedure

1. Mix all ingredients except egg and whey protein in a food processor to combine.
2. Add the egg and weigh protein and stir to combine.
3. Heat coconut oil over medium heat. Add heaped tablespoons of mixture to the pan, cook in batches for 2 mins each side or until browned.

Servings: 4 (8 fritters)

Total Time: 20 minutes

Nutrition Facts

Nutrition (per serving): 230 calories, 7.2g total fat, 127.8mg cholesterol, 198.1mg sodium, 618.4mg potassium, 5g carbohydrates, <1g fibre, 1.1g sugar, 34.7g protein.

DF, GF

Source

Thanks to Jane Allen at the Muffin Shop for donating this recipe. www.themuffinshop.com.au

Chicken Stir Fry

120 grams chicken thigh, cut into strips

1 cup green beans

3 asparagus spears, fresh, cut on diagonal

1 mushroom, field, sliced

1 tbsp super pesto

1 tsp extra virgin olive oil

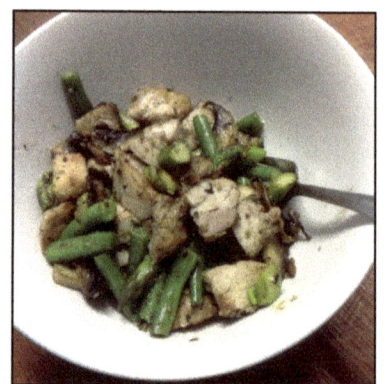

Procedure

1. Heat pan over medium heat, add the olive oil and sear the chicken.
2. Add remaining ingredients except pesto and stir-fry quickly until the vegetables are firm.
3. Stir pesto through in the last 5 minutes.

Servings: 1

Total Time: 20 minutes

Nutrition Facts

Nutrition (per serving): 292 calories, 15.1g total fat, 114mg cholesterol, 236.4mg sodium, 811.9mg potassium, 13.1g carbohydrates, 6.8g fibre, 5.4g sugar, 27.9g protein.

DF, GF

Recipe Tips

Delicious with Slendier pasta.

Chicken with Beetroot, Carrot, Apple and Ginger Salad

1 whole beetroot, raw, grated

3 whole carrots, grated

1 whole apple, grated

1 tbsp ginger, freshly grated (optional)

1/4 red cabbage, shredded

1 tsp olive oil

1 tbsp lemon juice

125 grams chicken breast, shredded

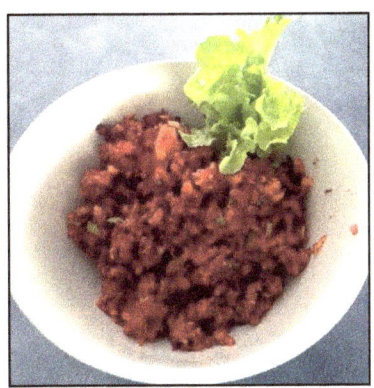

Procedure

1. Mix olive oil with lemon juice and set aside as the dressing.
2. Combined grated ingredients and drizzle with dressing.
3. Serve with shredded chicken.

Servings: 1

Total Time: 5 minutes

Nutrition Facts

Nutrition (per serving): 490 calories, 10.1g total fat, 106.3mg cholesterol, 354.1mg sodium, 1789.8mg potassium, 59.3g carbohydrates, 14.7g fibre, 35.8g sugar, 44.3g protein.

Source

Chimichurri Steak with Lemon Asparagus and Sweet Potato Chips

150 grams Topside steak
1 serve Sweet Potato Chips
1 tbsp Chimichurri
1 serve Asparagus with Lemon and Almonds
1 tomato, Roma type
1 small Spanish onion, whole

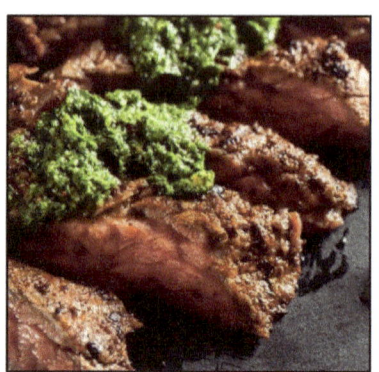

Procedure

1. Preheat oven to 200 degrees Celsius and put the Sweet Potato Chips into the oven, along with the whole onion (skin on).
2. When the chips are half cooked, slice tomato in half and add to tray.
3. Start preparing the Asparagus with Lemon and Almonds.
4. Heat a barbecue grill to medium heat; add steak and cook as desired.
5. Transfer steak to a plate and top with 1 tbsp Chimichurri.
6. Add oven-roasted vegetables, then asparagus, and serve.

Servings: 1

Total Time: 25 minutes

Nutrition Facts

Nutrition (per serving): 447 calories, 18.5g total fat, 61.5mg cholesterol, 251.6mg sodium, 865.5mg potassium, 35.2g carbohydrates, 8.2g fibre, 9.4g sugar, 38.5g protein.

DF, GF

Sweet potato is an excellent source of vitamin A and a low-GI form of carbohydrate.

Recipe Tips

Ensure chips are cut thinly. Order of cooking may need to be varied according to how you like your steak.

Indian Chicken

1/2 tsp coconut oil
1 onion, diced
1 garlic clove, crushed
1 tsp turmeric, ground
1 tsp mustard seed, yellow
1/2 tsp cumin seeds, ground
1 chili, red
3 tomatoes, diced
130 grams chicken breast, cut into strips
1 zucchini, cubed
3 tbsp coconut milk

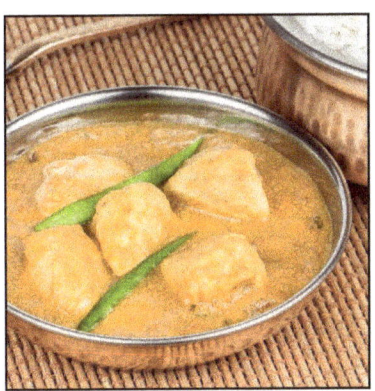

Procedure

1. Melt coconut oil in a pan over medium heat, sauté garlic and onion.
2. Add dried spices and chili; stir quickly for 15 seconds (mustard may pop).
3. Add chicken and brown.
4. Add tomatoes and coconut milk; stir well and cook through.
5. Serve with cauliflower rice.

Servings: 1

Total Time: 40 minutes

Nutrition Facts

Nutrition (per serving): 398 calories, 11.4g total fat, 83.2mg cholesterol, 199.9mg sodium, 2404.8mg potassium, 41.7g carbohydrates, 10.6g fibre, 24g sugar, 37.3g protein.

DF, GF

Mustard seeds are an excellent source of selenium and a good source of omega 3 fatty acids and manganese (www.whfoods.com). They are also a digestive aid.

Recipe Tips

Delicious with cauliflower rice and Indian Spinach.
Can be topped with 1 tsp crushed cashews (optional).

Indonesian Beef Stir Fry

1/2 tsp coconut oil
1 garlic clove, chopped
1/2 chilli, red
1 sprig coriander, finely chopped
250 grams beef steak, extra lean
4 stalks broccolini
1/2 red capsicum, cut into strips
1 tbsp lime juice
1 pinch stevia
2 tbsp coconut milk
1 tbsp fish sauce

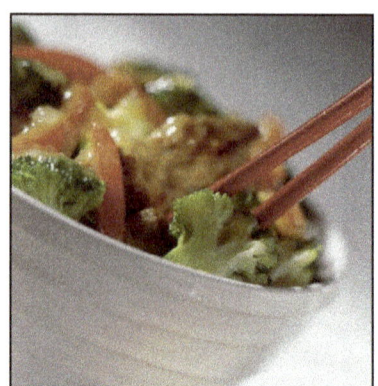

Procedure

1. Heat coconut oil over medium heat in a fry pan.
2. Add garlic, chili and coriander and stir to cook.
3. Add beef strips and sear.
4. Add chopped broccolini and capsicum (or carrot) and stir well.
5. Add lime juice, stevia, fish sauce and coconut milk.
6. Stir well to cook and slightly reduce sauce.
7. Serve on a bed of cauliflower rice.

Servings: 2

Total Time: 20 minutes

Nutrition Facts

Nutrition (per serving): 411 calories, 27.3g total fat, 106.3mg cholesterol, 813mg sodium, 1039.2mg potassium, 13g carbohydrates, 1.1g fibre, 2.6g sugar, 30.4g protein.

DF, GF

Coriander is known as an 'anti-diabetic' plant and is known for its anti-inflammatory and cholesterol-lowering properties (www.whfoods.com).

Mushroom Burgers

2 Portobello mushrooms, large, whole

1/2 tsp coconut oil

1 clove garlic

120 grams chicken breast (or firm tofu)

5 leaves sorrel

6 kale leaves, de-stemmed

1 sprig lemon thyme

1 serve Preserved Lemon Dressing

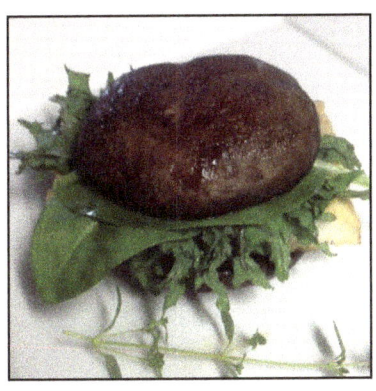

Procedure

1. Heat a fry pan over medium heat and melt coconut oil.
2. Remove mushroom stems, place open-side down and brown, approx. 4 minutes.
3. Add chicken breast or tofu to the pan and brown.

Servings: 1

Total Time: 15 minutes

Nutrition Facts

Nutrition (per serving): 353 calories, 21.7g total fat, 76.8mg cholesterol, 170.1mg sodium, 1153.4mg potassium, 11.5g carbohydrates, 2.3g fibre, <1g sugar, 31g protein.

Recipe Tips

* Vegetarian or vegan if using tofu instead of chicken

DF, GF, V, VG

About six species of mushrooms are known for their health promoting benefits, including improved immune function.

Nasi Goreng

1 serve Slendier pasta, fine
2 whole eggs, boiled
3 tbsp soy sauce or Bragg's
2 garlic cloves, crushed
1 inch ginger, freshly grated
4 shallots, coarsely chopped
120 grams chicken thigh, cut into strips
2 chili, red, chopped
1/2 cup coriander leaves
2 tbsp roasted peanuts

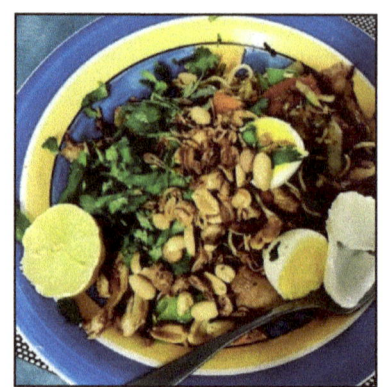

Procedure

1. Boil two eggs for 7 - 12 minutes until hard; drain and set aside.
2. Meanwhile, drain Slendier pasta and cover with boiling water; set aside.
3. Heat a non-stick pan to medium.
4. Quickly fry the peanuts, tossing or stirring to avoid burning. When browned, set aside.
5. Add garlic cloves, chili, ginger and shallots to the pan and fry until tender, then remove from pan.
6. Add chicken thigh strips to the pan; brown, then cook through.
7. Drain Slendier Pasta, add to the pan, stir well, heat through.
8. Add the soy sauce and stir quickly to combine and avoid sticking.
9. Transfer to a plate and add the boiled eggs and roasted peanuts.
10. Serve with a wedge of lime, fresh chili (if desired) and fresh coriander.

Servings: 2

Total Time: 45 minutes

Nutrition Facts

Nutrition (per serving): 251 calories, 12.7g total fat, 269.1mg cholesterol, 932.1mg sodium, 491.5mg potassium, 11.2g carbohydrates, 3.1g fibre, 4.3g sugar, 23.1g protein.

Pizza, low fat Chicken

1 serve Cauliflower Pizza or Tortilla Wrap, low fat

1 clove garlic, minced

2 tbsp tomato paste, salt-free

1 pinch coriander seeds

1 tbsp ricotta cheese, light

1 tbsp oregano leaves, chopped

100 grams chicken breast, cooked and chopped

5 broccoli florets, cut into small pieces

3 whole capers, drained (optional)

1 tomato, diced

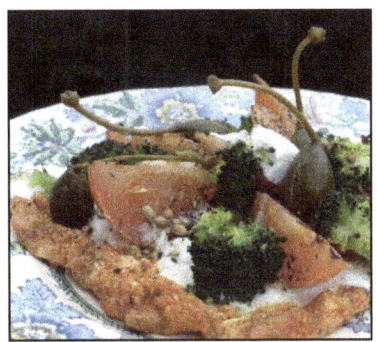

Procedure

1. Prepare the low-fat Cauliflower Pizza Base as per the recipe.
2. While the base is cooking, prepare the toppings.
3. Mix the garlic with tomato paste.
4. Remove cooked pizza base from the oven and top with the tomato paste mix.
5. Sprinkle herbs over the top.
6. Add onion, chicken, capsicum and extra light ricotta cheese (optional).
7. Return to oven and bake for 10 minutes.

Servings: 1

Yield: 2 pizzas

Total Time: 40 minutes

Nutrition Facts

Nutrition (per serving): 374 calories, 6.7g total fat, 89.8mg cholesterol, 543.1mg sodium, 1854.8mg potassium, 32g carbohydrates, 10.5g fibre, 14.4g sugar, 49.1g protein.

DF, GF

Pizza, Supreme

1 serve Cauliflower Pizza or Tortilla Wrap

1 clove garlic, minced

2 tbsp tomato paste, no added salt

1 tbsp parsley, finely chopped

1 tbsp oregano leaves, chopped

2 tbsp Parmesan cheese, grated

1 tbsp olives, sliced

1 rasher Short cut bacon, cut into squares

1/2 cup sweet potato, cubed and baked

1/4 avocado, cut into cubes

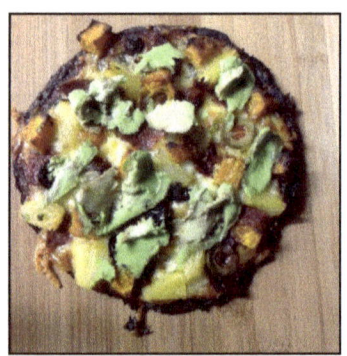

Procedure

1. Prepare the low-fat Cauliflower Pizza Base (see recipe).
2. Mix the garlic with tomato paste.
3. Remove cooked pizza base from oven, top with the tomato paste mix.
4. Sprinkle herbs and parmesan cheese over the top.
5. Top with remaining ingredients except avocado; bake 10 minutes.
6. Top with avocado and serve.

Servings: 1

Yield: 2 pizzas

Total Time: 40 minutes

Nutrition Facts

Nutrition (per serving): 511 calories, 24.5g total fat, 379.2mg cholesterol, 1026.2mg sodium, 2140.4mg potassium, 48.1g carbohydrates, 15.1g fibre, 20g sugar, 30.2g protein.

GF

Recipe Tips

Parmesan can be omitted or replaced with goat's cheese. Chopped kale or silverbeet leaves can be added in the last five minutes of cooking.

Satisfying Chicken Salad

80 grams chicken breast, cooked and chopped

100 grams sweet potato (cold), cooked and cubed

2 cups lettuce leaves, mixed types, shredded

2 sprigs parsley, chopped

2 sprigs mint leaves, chopped

1/4 avocado, cubed

1 tomato, Roma type, diced

1 tsp pumpkin seeds

1 tbsp Goat's feta, crumbled

1 tsp lemon juice

1 tsp balsamic vinegar

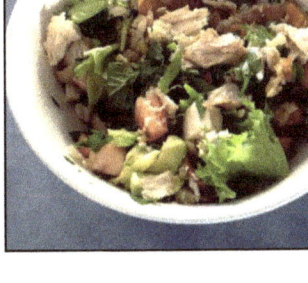

Procedure

1 Toss all ingredients in a large bowl to combine.

Servings: 1

Total Time: 10 minutes

Nutrition Facts

Nutrition (per serving): 395 calories, 14.1g total fat, 78.5mg cholesterol, 392.8mg sodium, 1539.3mg potassium, 35g carbohydrates, 9.7g fibre, 17g sugar, 33.9g protein.

GF

Silverbeet Salad Wraps

8 large silverbeet (chard) leaves, whole
1 cup carrot, grated
1 cup radish, grated
1 cup kale, finely chopped
1/2 cup snow peas, cut into strips
1 cup fresh coriander
1/2 cup avocado, mashed

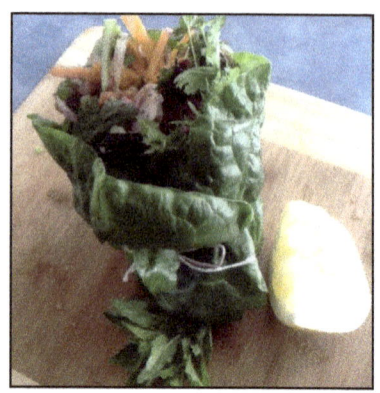

Procedure

1. Arrange 1/8th portion of each ingredient in the centre of a silverbeet or chard leaf.
2. Add any dressing you like, e.g. tahini, lemon and yoghurt.
3. Fold the bottom of the leaf up, then fold across the side where the stem is thickest.
4. Roll the stuffed silverbeet leaf up, toward the tip of the leaf.
5. Tie with a piece of kitchen twine and refrigerate until ready to use.

Servings: 4

Yield: 8 wraps

Total Time: 10 minutes

Nutrition Facts

Nutrition (per serving): 76 calories, 3.2g total fat, 0mg cholesterol, 243.2mg sodium, 713.6mg potassium, 10.9g carbohydrates, 4.3g fibre, 3.4g sugar, 3.5g protein.

DF, GF, V, VG

Recipe Tips

Chard leaves are often softer and more pliable than silverbeet. Soft lettuce leaves may be used instead.

Soft Lamb Tortillas

1/2 Spanish onion, finely chopped

1 garlic clove, crushed

80 grams lamb roast (lean, leftover)

1 tbsp Salsa

1 Cauliflower Tortilla - Low Fat

1 sprig coriander leaves, roughly chopped

1 sprig oregano leaves, diced

1 cup lettuce leaves, mixed types, torn

1 tbsp Guacamole

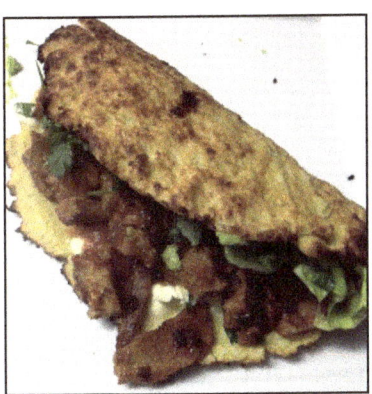

Procedure

1. Heat a fry pan over medium heat.
2. Brown the onion and garlic.
3. Add the leftover lamb and salsa; stir to combine and heat through (add a little water to avoid sticking if required).
4. Place a warm Cauliflower Tortilla on a plate.
5. Top with lamb mix, cheese, coriander and lettuce.
6. Serve immediately.

Servings: 1

Total Time: 40 minutes

Nutrition Facts

Nutrition (per serving): 572 calories, 25g total fat, 84mg cholesterol, 996.3mg sodium, 2424.4mg potassium, 52.5g carbohydrates, 19.5g fibre, 20.2g sugar, 41.6g protein.

DF, GF, V

Grass-fed lamb is an excellent source of vitamin B12 and a significant source of omega 3 fatty acids, which are beneficial for heart health and lowering inflammation. It is also a good source of zinc which is essential for immune health.

Spaghetti Squash Bolognaise

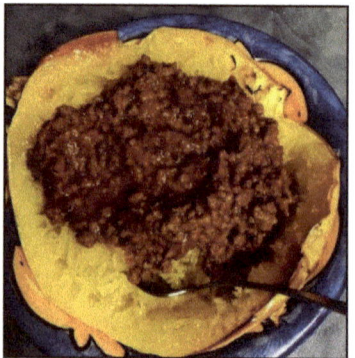

1 tsp olive oil
1 clove garlic, minced
30 grams onions, chopped
120 grams lean veal & pork mince
75 grams tomato paste
1 whole tomato, diced
1 sprig parsley, finely chopped
1 sprig oregano leaves, crushed
1 sprig basil, chopped
1/2 cup water (if desired)
1/2 medium spaghetti squash

Procedure

1. Preheat the oven to 200 degrees C.
2. Place the squash cut side down on a lightly oiled baking tray; roast for 30 minutes.
3. Meanwhile, heat a non-stick pan to medium heat.
4. Add the oil, garlic and onions, sauté until lightly browned.
5. Add the veal and pork mince and sauté until evenly browned.
6. Add tomato paste, the chopped tomato and up to 1/2 cup of water to obtain a good consistency.
7. Cover; simmer gently for 10 - 12 minutes to reduce the sauce.
8. Add chopped fresh herbs in the last three minutes of cooking.
9. Season with salt and pepper if desired.
10. Remove squash from the oven and transfer to a bowl.
11. Use a fork to tease out the spaghetti from the squash.
12. Add the bolognaise sauce and serve immediately.
13. Note; you can replace the spaghetti squash with zucchini noodles or cubes of roasted pumpkin if you prefer.

Servings: 1

Total Time: 40 minutes

Nutrition Facts

Nutrition (per serving): 340 calories, 10.5g total fat, 70.8mg cholesterol, 175.7mg sodium, 1630.9mg potassium, 36.1g carbohydrates, 8.1g fibre, 18g sugar, 31.3g protein.

Spring Tuna Salad

1 cup baby spinach

1/2 cup snow peas, chopped in half

2 sticks celery, chopped

1 spring onion, finely chopped

1/4 whole avocado, diced

185 grams tuna in oil

1 tbsp lemon juice or white wine vinegar

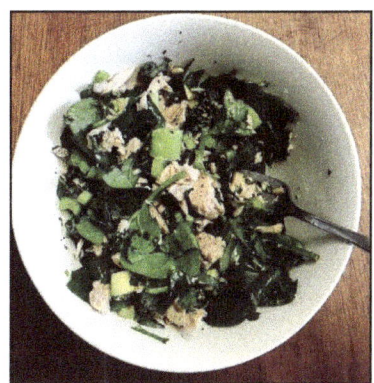

Procedure

1. Mix salad ingredients together.
2. Stir through canned tuna.
3. Drizzle lemon juice over the top, season to taste and serve immediately.

Servings: 1

Total Time: 5 minutes

Nutrition Facts

Nutrition (per serving): 454 calories, 21.1g total fat, 30.8mg cholesterol, 708.4mg sodium, 1096.5mg potassium, 12.1g carbohydrates, 6.3g fibre, 3.9g sugar, 53.4g protein.

Summer Stir Fry

150 grams chicken breasts, sliced into strips

1 zucchini, thinly sliced

1 button squash, thinly sliced

1 carrot, cut into sticks

3 asparagus spears, large, fresh

4 kale leaves, de-stemmed and torn

1 cup green beans

1/2 tsp coconut oil

1 tsp balsamic vinegar

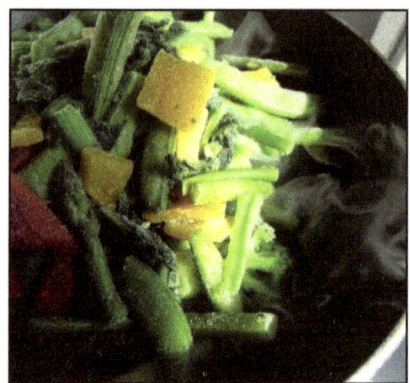

Procedure

1. Heat coconut oil over medium heat in a frypan.
2. Sear the strips so they are browned and cook through. Set aside.
3. Add vegetables and stir to coat evenly with oil.
4. Cook for 5 minutes (firm).
5. Return chicken to the pan and stir through balsamic vinegar and serve.

Servings: 1

Total Time: 15 minutes

Nutrition Facts

Nutrition (per serving): 374 calories, 8.6g total fat, 96mg cholesterol, 297mg sodium, 2548.8mg potassium, 36.8g carbohydrates, 10.3g fibre, 19.4g sugar, 43.5g protein.

Recipe Tips

Serve with grilled chicken or fish.

* Low FODMAP if the asparagus is omitted.

Surf and Turf with Spicy Avo Sauce

200 grams Topside grass-fed steak, extra lean

100 grams smoked salmon

2 serve Spicy Avocado Sauce

1 serve cucumber, thinly sliced

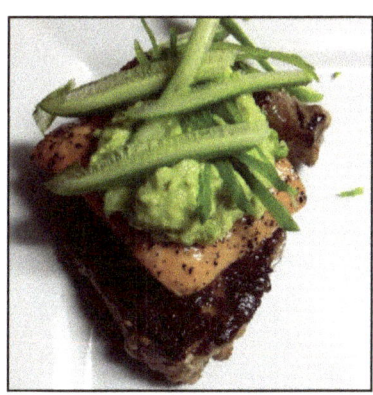

Procedure

1. Heat the barbecue and grill the steak to your liking.
2. Top with hot smoked salmon in the last 3 minutes of cooking, to heat the salmon through.
3. Remove from the grill and plate the steak and fish.
4. Top with Spicy Avocado Sauce and cucumber sticks.

Servings: 2

Total Time: 20 minutes

Nutrition Facts

Nutrition (per serving): 355 calories, 21.2g total fat, 41mg cholesterol, 225.9mg sodium, 295.4mg potassium, 6g carbohydrates, 4.1g fibre, <1g sugar, 30.5g protein.

DF, GF

Recipe Tips

Delicious with a green salad.

Tasty Beef Burgers

1/2 onion, finely diced

1 garlic clove, crushed

75 grams cauliflower, grated

400 grams beef mince, extra lean

1 tbsp tapenade, pure olive

1 tbsp semi-dried tomatoes, finely diced (dry, not in oil)

1 tbsp oregano leaves, crushed

1 tbsp basil leaves, chopped

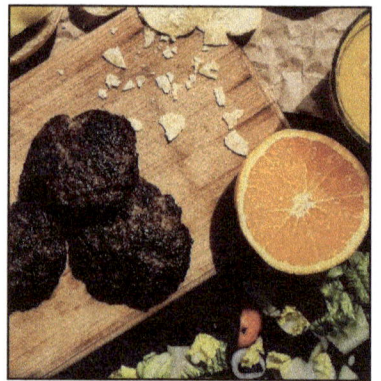

Procedure

1. Fry onion, garlic and cauliflower in a non-stick pan over medium heat.
2. Transfer to a bowl; combine with remaining ingredients and mix well.
3. Shape mixture into four large or eight small patties.
4. Fry patties in a non-stick pan until cooked through, flipping to brown.
5. Serve with a side salad.

Servings: 4

Total Time: 35 minutes

Nutrition Facts

Nutrition (per serving): 177 calories, 7.6g total fat, 62mg cholesterol, 223.5mg sodium, 464.8mg potassium, 3.9g carbohydrates, 1.1g fibre, 1.3g sugar, 22.2g protein.

DF, GF

Recipe Tips

Tapenade is pureed olive paste.

Tuna Bolognaise

1/2 tsp coconut oil

1 onion, finely diced

1 garlic clove, crushed

2 stalks celery or fennel, finely diced

300 grams tuna, (fresh if possible), flaked

2 tbsp tomato puree

1 can tomatoes, diced

1 pinch Himalayan salt

1 sprig oregano, chopped

1 sprig parsley, finely chopped

1 serve Slendier fettuccini

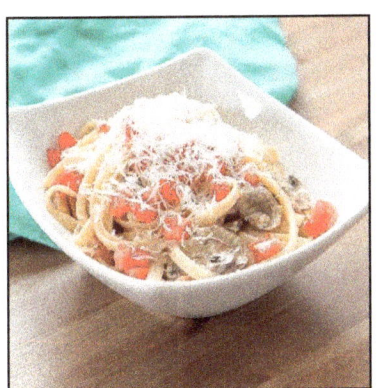

Procedure

1. Heat oil in a pan on medium heat.
2. Fry onion, garlic and celery for 3 - 5 minutes.
3. Add flaked tuna and stir in quickly.
4. Add tomato paste and diced tomatoes, stir well and reduce heat.
5. Simmer for 15 minutes until the sauce has thickened.
6. Add salt and fresh herbs, stir well and cook for a further 5 minutes.
7. Serve with Slendier fettuccini and garnish with cherry tomatoes.

Servings: 2

Total Time: 35 minutes

Nutrition Facts

Nutrition (per serving): 260 calories, 6g total fat, 63mg cholesterol, 836.3mg sodium, 839.1mg potassium, 12.3g carbohydrates, 5.6g fibre, 6.7g sugar, 37.5g protein.

DF, GF

5 Salad and Vegetables

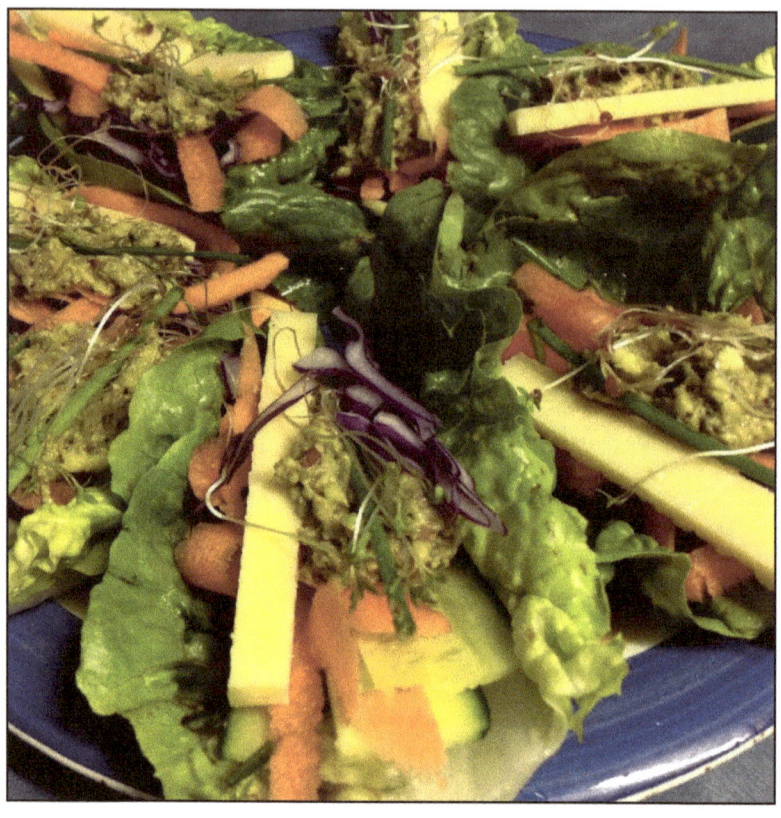

Asparagus with Lemon and Almonds

4 asparagus spears, large, fresh

1/2 tsp lemon zest

1/2 tsp extra virgin olive oil

1 tsp almonds, chopped

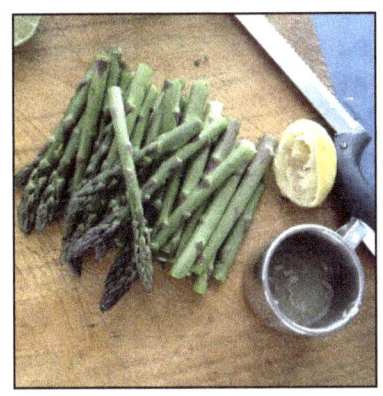

Procedure

1. Heat a non-stick pan over medium heat and toast the almonds until lightly golden.
2. Remove almonds from pan.
3. Add olive oil to the pan and then add asparagus; toss to combine.
4. Lightly brown the asparagus spears, turning regularly.
5. Add the lemon zest in the last minute of cooking.
6. Transfer to a serving dish and top with toasted almonds.

Servings: 1

Total Time: 15 minutes

Nutrition Facts

Nutrition (per serving): 48 calories, 3.3g total fat, 0mg cholesterol, 1.7mg sodium, 177.2mg potassium, 3.7g carbohydrates, 2g fibre, 1.6g sugar, 2.2g protein.

DF, GF, V, VG

Asparagus is an excellent source of vitamin K, folate, copper, vitamin B1, selenium, vitamin B2, vitamin C and vitamin E (www.whfoods.com).

Recipe Tips

Delicious with a lean grilled steak or as an accompaniment to grilled fish.

Beetslaw

1 medium beetroot, washed, topped and tailed
1 whole pink lady apple, grated
5 medium kale leaves, shredded
1/4 small cabbage (any kind), shredded
1/2 medium carrot, grated
2 tbsp lemon juice
1 tbsp sunflower oil

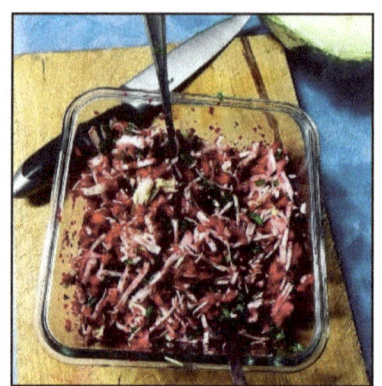

Procedure

1. Mix lemon juice and sunflower oil together and lightly season.
2. Toss all remaining ingredients to thoroughly combine.
3. Drizzle the slaw with dressing and serve immediately.

Servings: 1

Total Time: 5 minutes

Nutrition Facts

Nutrition (per serving): 325 calories, 14.9g total fat, 0mg cholesterol, 133.6mg sodium, 1044.3mg potassium, 46.7g carbohydrates, 9.3g fibre, 27.4g sugar, 6g protein.

Recipe Tips

* Low FODMAP if one small celery stalk used

Carrot and Hazelnut Salad

1 medium carrot, finely grated

1/2 Spanish onion, finely chopped

1 tbsp hazelnuts, roasted, chopped

1 cup mint leaves, chopped

1/2 tsp coriander, ground

1/2 tsp cumin seeds, ground

1/2 tsp fennel seeds, crushed

1 tsp extra virgin olive oil

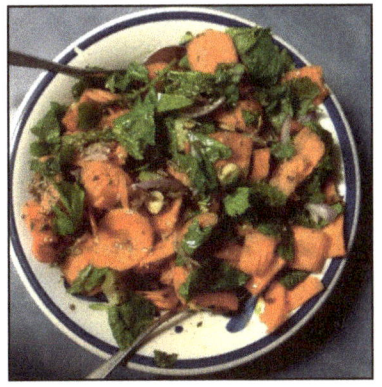

Procedure

1. Toss carrot, onion, mint and hazelnuts.
2. Mix spices with olive oil and drizzle over salad.

Servings: 1

Total Time: 5 minutes

Nutrition Facts

Nutrition (per serving): 174 calories, 12g total fat, 0mg cholesterol, 65.8mg sodium, 628mg potassium, 15.8g carbohydrates, 5.6g fibre, 3.4g sugar, 4.9g protein.

DF, GF, V, VG

Hazelnuts are an excellent source of manganese, vitamin E and thiamin.

Recipe Tips

A great side dish for grilled lean lamb chops.

Carrot and Kale Salad

1 medium carrot, finely grated

1 cup kale, finely chopped

2 cups lettuce leaves, mixed types, torn

1 sprig coriander leaves, roughly chopped (optional)

1 serve Tahini Lemon Dressing

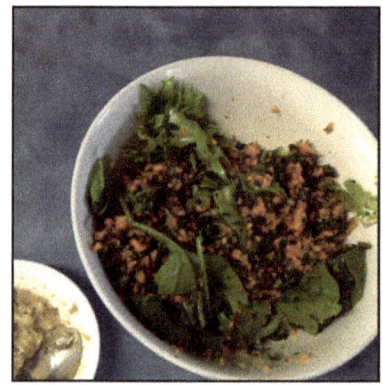

Procedure

1. Combine ingredients and toss well with two forks.
2. Serve with Tahini Lemon Dressing and your favourite lean protein.

Servings: 1

Total Time: 5 minutes

Nutrition Facts

Nutrition (per serving): 90 calories, 2.4g total fat, 0mg cholesterol, 78.2mg sodium, 831.1mg potassium, 15.5g carbohydrates, 3.6g fibre, 4.1g sugar, 5.6g protein.

DF, FOD, GF, V, VG

Coleslaw

100 grams cabbage (any kind), shredded

50 grams silverbeet (or chard) or mixed herbs, raw, chopped

1 carrot, grated

2 celery stalks, diced

1 tbsp parsley leaves

1/2 tsp pine nuts, toasted

1/2 tsp pepitas

1 tsp mayonnaise, whole egg

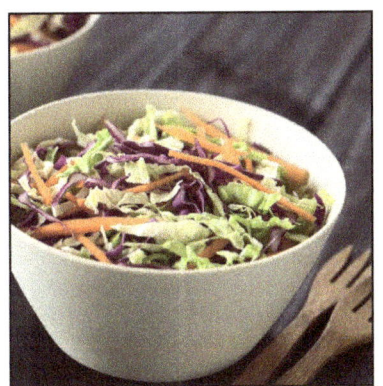

Procedure

1 Toss ingredients well and serve immediately.

Servings: 1

Total Time: 5 minutes

Nutrition Facts

Nutrition (per serving): 119 calories, 3.8g total fat, 1.3mg cholesterol, 289.4mg sodium, 893.1mg potassium, 19.8g carbohydrates, 7.3g fibre, 9.7g sugar, 4.3g protein.

DF, FOD, GF, V

Recipe Tips

* Low FODMAP if one small celery stalk used

Cucumber and Fennel Salad

1/2 Lebanese cucumber, sliced
3 stalks celery, finely chopped
1/2 fennel bulb, shredded
1 shallot, finely chopped
2 chives, finely chopped
2 tbsp Greek yoghurt, low fat
1 tsp lemon juice
1 pinch stevia

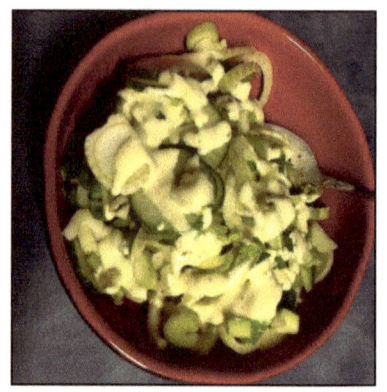

Procedure

1. Toss chopped vegetables in a serving bowl.
2. Mix yoghurt with lemon juice and stevia, drizzle over salad.

Servings: 2

Total Time: 5 minutes

Nutrition Facts

Nutrition (per serving): 203 calories, 1.7g total fat, 0mg cholesterol, 120.9mg sodium, 1196mg potassium, 43.2g carbohydrates, 9.9g fibre, 19.7g sugar, 7.9g protein.

DF, FOD, GF, V

* Low FODMAP if one stalk of celery used, lactose-free yoghurt used and no shallots.

Eggplant Parmigiana

1 eggplant, sliced into rounds (1cm thick)
1 garlic clove, crushed
1 onion, diced
2 tbsp tomato paste
1 tomato, diced
1 tsp oregano leaves, crushed
1 tsp basil leaves, chopped
1 tsp parsley, finely chopped

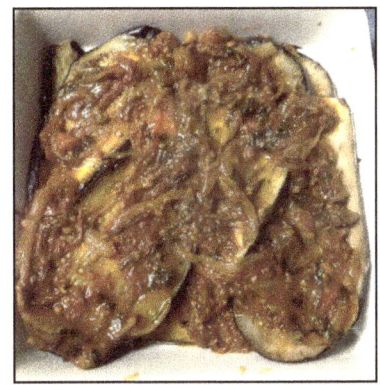

Procedure

1. Salt the eggplant slices and set aside.
2. Stir-fry the garlic and onion in a small fry pan until transparent.
3. Add the tomato paste and fresh tomato, plus a little water to make a thick sauce.
4. Add the herbs, stir well until combined and warmed.
5. Rinse the eggplant and lightly cook under the griller, until just soft.
6. Transfer the eggplant to a baking dish.
7. Top with the onion/tomato mix.
8. Bake at 180 degrees Celsius for 15 minutes or until cooked.

Servings: 2

Total Time: 30 minutes

Nutrition Facts

Nutrition (per serving): 111 calories, <1g total fat, 0mg cholesterol, 20.5mg sodium, 953.8mg potassium, 25.5g carbohydrates, 9.6g fibre, 14.4g sugar, 4.4g protein.

DF, GF, V, VG

Recipe Tips

Delicious with lean beef, lamb or kangaroo.

Eggplant, Tomato and Feta Salad (Grumpy and Sweetheart's)

1 tsp olive oil (marinade)
1 clove garlic, minced (marinade)
1/2 tsp Italian herbs (marinade)
1/2 tsp chili flakes (marinade)
1 tsp lemon zest (marinade)
100 grams feta, marinated, cubed
1 large eggplant, chopped
1 punnet cherry tomatoes
1 red capsicum, diced
4 cloves garlic, unpeeled
2 tbsp extra virgin olive oil
2 tbsp mint leaves, chopped
2 tbsp chives, snipped
1/4 cup olive oil (dressing)
1/2 cup balsamic vinegar (dressing)
1 tsp Dijon mustard (dressing)
1 tsp honey (dressing)
1 pinch salt (dressing)

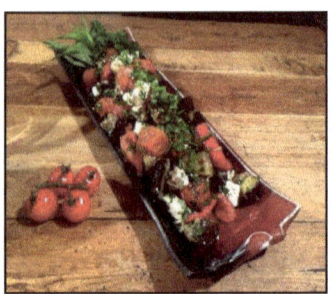

Procedure

1. Combine marinade ingredients and add cubed feta. Set aside.
2. Combine eggplant, tomatoes, capsicum, olive oil and garlic on a baking tray. Season to taste.
3. Bake until eggplant is lightly golden, about 15 minutes.
4. Combine the dressing ingredients in a small jar.
5. Transfer the warm vegetables to a serving bowl.
6. Squeeze roasted garlic into balsamic dressing; blend with a stick mixer.
7. Top the warm vegetables with the marinated feta and drizzle with dressing.

Servings: 4

Total Time: 30 minutes

Nutrition Facts

Nutrition (per serving): 351 calories, 27.3g total fat, 22.3mg cholesterol, 389.5mg sodium, 566.5mg potassium, 21.8g carbohydrates, 5.7g fibre, 13.7g sugar, 6.2g protein.

DF, V

Recipe Tips

Delicious with grilled chicken or fish.

Source

Source: Thanks to Elizabeth Connell of Grumpy and Sweetheart's for donating this recipe.

Greek Kale Salad

1 cup spinach leaves

1 cup kale, finely chopped

1 capsicum, red, finely chopped

1/4 Spanish onion, very finely chopped

4 olives, sliced

1 tbsp avocado, diced

1 tsp oregano leaves, diced

1 tbsp basil leaves, chopped

1 tbsp balsamic vinegar or 1 tsp. fresh lemon juice

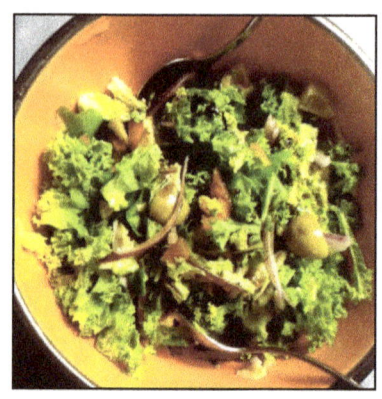

Procedure

1. Toss spinach, kale, capsicum, onion, olives, basil, avocado and oregano.
2. Top with balsamic vinegar or lemon juice.

Servings: 1

Total Time: 5 minutes

Nutrition Facts

Nutrition (per serving): 156 calories, 5.3g total fat, 0mg cholesterol, 214.2mg sodium, 911.3mg potassium, 23.5g carbohydrates, 6.2g fibre, 8.7g sugar, 6.1g protein.

DF, GF, V, VG

Recipe Tips

Serve with a lean protein.

Indian Spinach

4 cups silverbeet (or chard), raw, chopped

1 spring onion, finely chopped

1 tsp turmeric, ground or grated

1 garlic clove, crushed

1 tsp lemongrass, minced

1/2 tsp garam masala

1/2 tsp coriander seed, ground

1/2 tsp cardamom

3 tbsp Greek yoghurt (low-fat or regular)

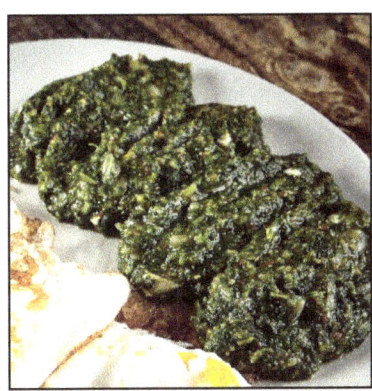

Procedure

1. Dry-fry the spring onion and spices in a fry pan over medium heat.
2. Add the silverbeet and 1 tbsp water; stir for 5 minutes until silverbeet wilts.
3. Add yoghurt and stir through.
4. Sprinkle with chilli flakes if desired.

Servings: 1

Total Time: 15 minutes

Nutrition Facts

Nutrition (per serving): 116 calories, 4.1g total fat, 0mg cholesterol, 344.7mg sodium, 690.6mg potassium, 15.6g carbohydrates, 3.9g fibre, 7.1g sugar, 7g protein.

FOD, GF, V

* Low FODMAP if lactose-free yoghurt is used.

Recipe Tips

Fermentation bubbles are a normal part of the fermentation process. Remove any surface mould if it appears. Sauerkraut stores for up to three months in the refrigerator.

Roasted Sweet Potato and Fig Salad with Balsamic Glaze

1 medium sweet potato, cut into thin wedges

1 tsp coconut oil

4 black figs, trimmed and cut in half

3 tbsp balsamic vinegar

3 tbsp water

1 tbsp maple syrup

1 small red chili, finely sliced

3 spring onions, chopped

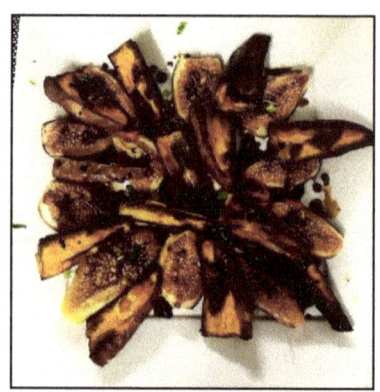

Procedure

1. Massage slightly-melted coconut oil into sweet potato sticks.
2. Place on a tray lined with baking paper.
3. Bake in a pre-heated oven at 200 degrees C for 30 minutes, until browned and cooked through.
4. Add balsamic, water and maple syrup to a small saucepan and bring to the boil; simmer until reduced and slightly thick.
5. Meanwhile, place the fig halves on a baking tray and place under the grill 5 - 7 minutes until golden on top.
6. Finely slice the chili and add to the balsamic reduction.
7. Arrange the sweet potato chips and fig halves on a plate and sprinkle with chopped spring onions.
8. Drizzle with balsamic chili glaze and serve.
9. Delicious with marinated beef or lamb.

Servings: 2

Total Time: 30 minutes

Nutrition Facts

Nutrition (per serving): 213 calories, 2.7g total fat, 0mg cholesterol, 49.9mg sodium, 636.5mg potassium, 46.8g carbohydrates, 5.8g fibre, 31.1g sugar, 2.7g protein.

Shaved Fennel and Kale Salad

1 large fennel bulb, shredded

1 cup kale, torn

1 tsp preserved lemon or lemon zest, finely chopped

1 tbsp parmesan, grated

1 sprig thyme

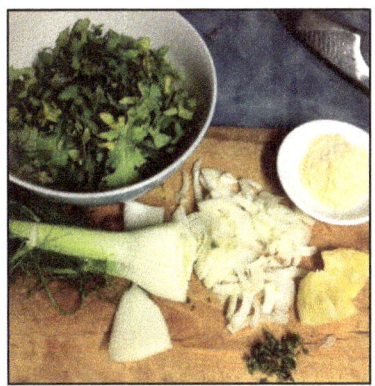

Procedure

1. Toss fennel and kale.
2. Sprinkle with preserved lemon, thyme and parmesan.

Servings: 2

Total Time: 5 minutes

Nutrition Facts

Nutrition (per serving): 42 calories, 1.1g total fat, 2.2mg cholesterol, 73.8mg sodium, 354.9mg potassium, 6.8g carbohydrates, 1.7g fibre, <1g sugar, 3g protein.

FOD, GF, V, VG

Fennel is used for various digestive problems including heartburn, intestinal gas, bloating, and colic in infants (www.webmd.com).

Recipe Tips

A delicious topping for steaks, goulash or casseroles.

Simple Avo and Pea Salad

1 whole avocado, peeled and diced

2 cups mixed lettuce leaves

1 cup snow peas or snap peas, tailed and cut in half

1 tbsp lemon juice

salt and pepper to taste

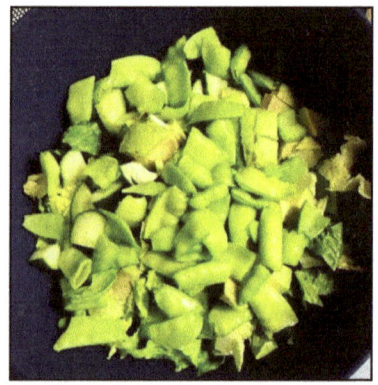

Procedure

1. Toss the avocado, peas and lettuce well.
2. Drizzle with lemon juice and season to taste.
3. Serve with beef or lamb.

Servings: 2

Total Time: 5 minutes

Nutrition Facts

Nutrition (per serving): 182 calories, 14.9g total fat, 0mg cholesterol, 158.8mg sodium, 646.8mg potassium, 12.6g carbohydrates, 8.4g fibre, 2.1g sugar, 3.5g protein.

Sweet Potato Chips

100 grams sweet potato, cut into 1cm-thick sticks

1 tsp coconut oil

1/2 tsp sumac (optional)

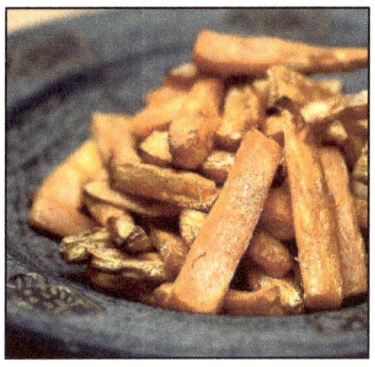

Procedure

1. Massage slightly-melted coconut oil into sweet potato sticks.
2. Place on a tray lined with baking paper.
3. Season to taste and/or sprinkle with sumac.
4. Bake in a pre-heated oven at 200 degrees C for 20 minutes, until browned.

Servings: 1

Total Time: 30 minutes

Nutrition Facts

Nutrition (per serving): 130 calories, 4.8g total fat, 0mg cholesterol, 139mg sodium, 337mg potassium, 21g carbohydrates, 3g fibre, 4.2g sugar, 1.7g protein.

DF, FOD, GF, V, VG

Tabbouleh

3 sprigs mint leaves, chopped

3 sprigs parsley, chopped

1 small cucumber, Lebanese with skin, diced

8 cherry tomatoes, quartered

1/2 tsp coconut oil

3/4 cup cauliflower, grated

1 tsp preserved lemon or lemon zest, finely chopped

1 pinch Himalayan salt

1 pinch black pepper freshly ground

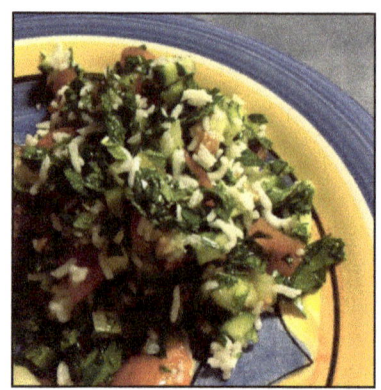

Procedure

1. Toss the mint, parsley, cucumber and cherry tomatoes.
2. Heat oil in a pan over medium heat, add grated cauliflower, stir fry until lightly browned, then set aside to cool.
3. Toss cooked cauliflower and finely chopped preserved lemon (or 1 tbsp lemon juice) through the salad.
4. Season with salt and pepper.

Servings: 1

Total Time: 15 minutes

Nutrition Facts

Nutrition (per serving): 127 calories, 3.8g total fat, 0mg cholesterol, 47.8mg sodium, 1065mg potassium, 23.6g carbohydrates, 5.6g fibre, 6.6g sugar, 5.3g protein.

DF, GF, V, VG

Recipe Tips

Delicious with grilled lamb or chicken.

Winter Greens Salad

1 cup watercress leaves

2 leaves silverbeet (chard), raw, finely chopped

8 leaves kale, finely chopped

2 tbsp parsley, chopped

2 tbsp marjoram leaves

2 radishes, cut into strips

1 tsp preserved lemon or lemon zest, finely chopped

1 tbsp apple cider vinegar

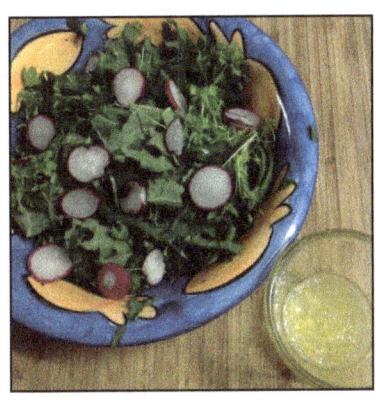

Procedure

1. Mix salad leaves and radish together to combine.
2. Mix preserved lemon with vinegar and splash over salad.
3. Serve with your favourite protein.

Servings: 2

Total Time: 5 minutes

Nutrition Facts

Nutrition (per serving): 53 calories, <1g total fat, 0mg cholesterol, 140.3mg sodium, 631.4mg potassium, 9.5g carbohydrates, 1.8g fibre, <1g sugar, 4.5g protein.

DF, FOD, GF, V, VG

6 Sauces and Sides

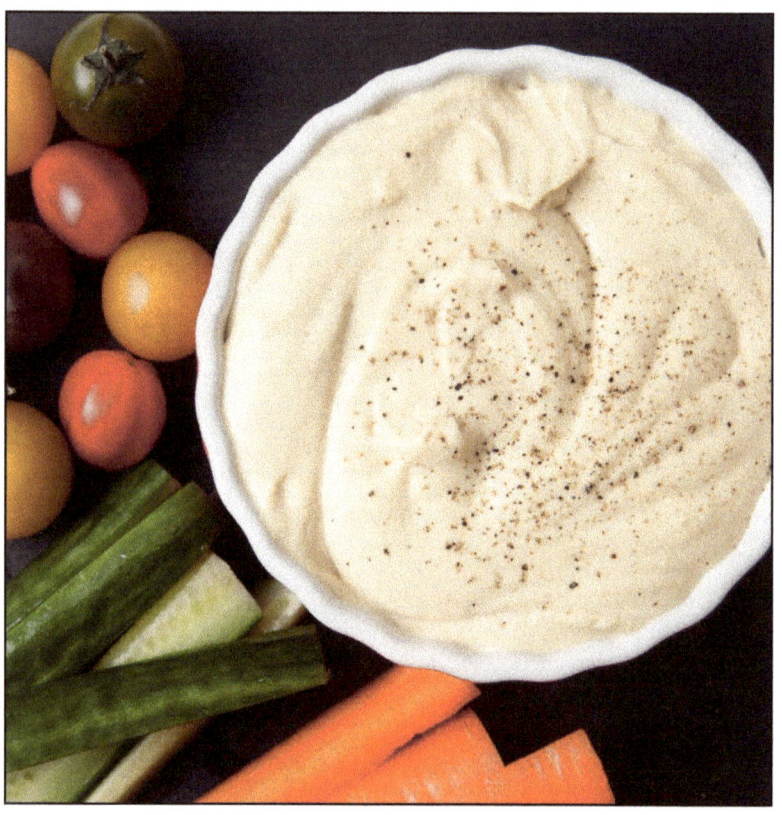

Chimichurri

1 garlic clove, crushed
1 cup parsley leaves, finely chopped
1/2 cup oregano leaves, finely chopped
1/4 cup extra virgin olive oil
1 tbsp lemon juice
1/2 tsp cumin seeds
1 pinch chilli flakes
1 pinch Himalayan salt
1/2 tsp cracked black pepper
1 tsp vinegar

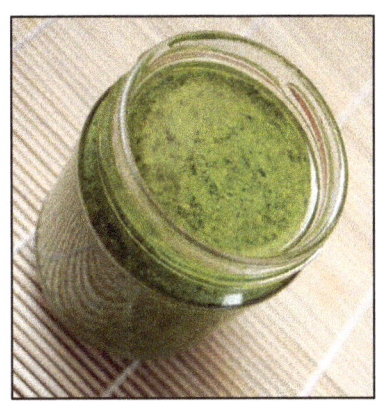

Procedure

1. Combine the finely chopped garlic, parsley and oregano.
2. Drizzle over olive oil and add remaining ingredients.
3. Marinate overnight (preferable) or serve immediately.

Servings: 10

Total Time: 15 minutes

Nutrition Facts

Nutrition (per serving): 56 calories, 5.5g total fat, 0mg cholesterol, 7mg sodium, 62.2mg potassium, 1.4g carbohydrates, 1.2g fibre, <1g sugar, <1g protein.

DF, GF, V, VG

Recipe Tips

A delicious topping for steak, chicken, salads or hot vegetables. Can be used as a dip.
This is an Argentinian sauce to be served with barbecued meat.

Gremolata

1 cup parsley, finely chopped

1 garlic clove, crushed

1 tbsp lemon zest, finely grated

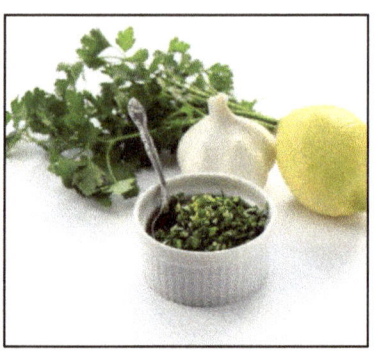

Procedure

1. Blitz ingredients in a food processor.
2. Use as a dressing for your favourite salad.

Servings: 2

Total Time: 5 minutes

Nutrition Facts

Nutrition (per serving): 14 calories, <1g total fat, 0mg cholesterol, 17.2mg sodium, 177mg potassium, 2.9g carbohydrates, 1.3g fibre, <1g sugar, 1g protein.

DF, GF, V, VG

Recipe Tips

A delicious topping for steaks, goulash or casseroles.

Preserved Lemon Dressing

1 piece preserved lemon
100 ml white wine vinegar
100 ml extra virgin olive oil

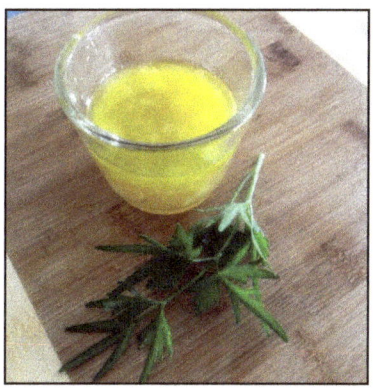

Procedure

1. Chop preserved lemon finely, mix all ingredients well.
2. Keeps in the refrigerator for up to 3 weeks.

Servings: 6

Total Time: 5 minutes

Nutrition Facts

Nutrition (per serving): 138 calories, 15.2g total fat, 0mg cholesterol, <1mg sodium, 22.3mg potassium, 1.4g carbohydrates, <1g fibre, 0g sugar, <1g protein.

DF, FOD, GF, V, VG

Raspberry Jam

60 grams raspberries

1 tsp chia seeds

1 pinch stevia (if desired, to taste)

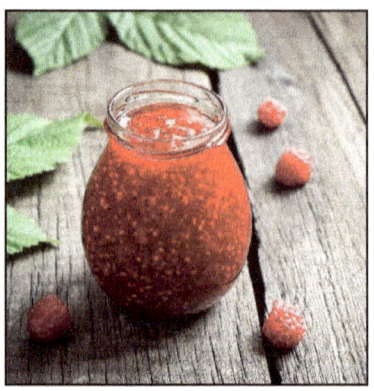

Procedure

1. Puree ingredients and transfer to a small jar or serving dish.
2. Keeps in the refrigerator for up to one week.

Servings: 2

Total Time: 5 minutes

Nutrition Facts

Nutrition (per serving): 20 calories, <1g total fat, 0mg cholesterol, <1mg sodium, 49.4mg potassium, 4g carbohydrates, 2.3g fibre, 1.3g sugar, <1g protein.

DF, FOD, GF, V, VG

Keep fresh raspberries refrigerated and consume within 1 – 2 days of purchase for maximum antioxidant benefits.

Spicy Avocado Sauce

1/2 avocado
2 tbsp almond milk
1/2 tsp Wasabi paste
1 pinch Himalayan salt

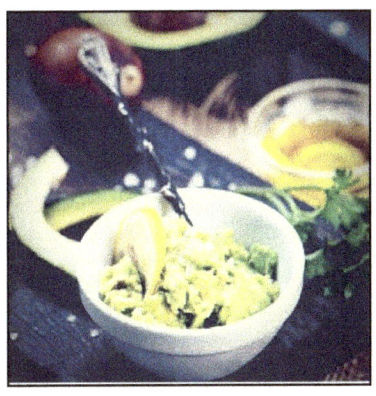

Procedure

1. Mash ingredients well.
2. A delicious topping for grilled steak or seafood.

Servings: 2

Yield: 2 serves

Total Time: 5 minutes

Nutrition Facts

Nutrition (per serving): 116 calories, 11g total fat, 0mg cholesterol, 9.8mg sodium, 289.3mg potassium, 5.4g carbohydrates, 3.8g fibre, <1g sugar, 1.4g protein.

DF, GF, V, VG

One cup of avocado or avocado oil, added to a salad of romaine lettuce, spinach and carrots, increases the absorption of carotenoids by 200 – 400% (www.whfoods.com).

Super Pesto

1 cup parsley leaves
1 cup basil leaves
1 cup oregano leaves
50 grams macadamia nuts or almonds
1 tbsp olive oil
1 garlic clove
1 small chili (optional)
1/2 tsp Himalayan salt

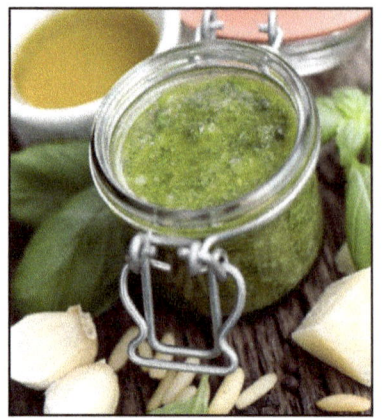

Procedure

1. Blend all ingredients until chunky and well mixed.
2. Refrigerate in a well-sealed jar.

Servings: 10

Total Time: 5 minutes

Nutrition Facts

Nutrition (per serving): 62 calories, 5.3g total fat, 0mg cholesterol, 120.9mg sodium, 121.7mg potassium, 2.9g carbohydrates, 2.6g fibre, <1g sugar, 1.1g protein.

DF, GF, V, VG

Parsley is an excellent source of vitamins K, C and A, folate and iron (www.whfood.com).

Recipe Tips

Enjoy stirred into soups, on top of grilled steak, or stirred through vegetables or salads.
Keeps for up to 3 weeks.

Source

Source: Image: Christianjung | Dreamstime.com

Tahini Lemon Dressing

1 tsp preserved lemon or lemon zest, finely chopped

1/2 tsp tahini

1/4 tsp cumin seeds, ground

1/4 tsp rosemary, fresh, finely chopped

1 tbsp water

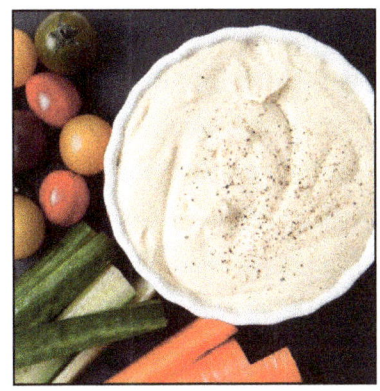

Procedure

1. Mix all ingredients well with a teaspoon.
2. Drizzle over your favourite salad.

Servings: 1

Total Time: 5 minutes

Nutrition Facts

Nutrition (per serving): 17 calories, 1.3g total fat, 0mg cholesterol, 3.3mg sodium, 24.3mg potassium, 1.2g carbohydrates, <1g fibre, <1g sugar, <1g protein.

DF, FOD, GF, V, VG

Recipe Tips

Un-hulled tahini is darker, and has a stronger taste and higher fibre content, than hulled tahini.

7 Snacks

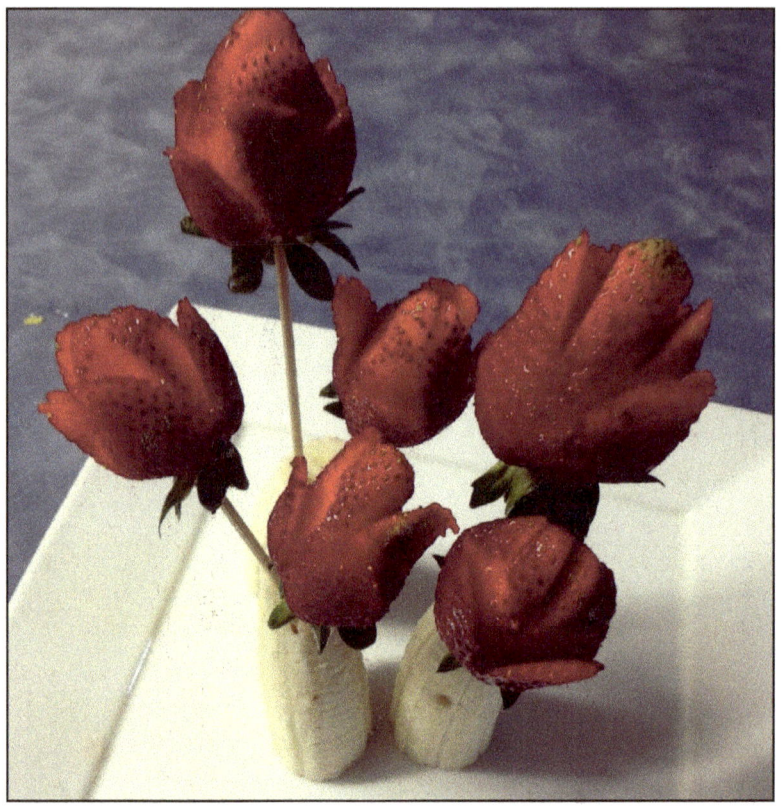

Christmas Balls

100 grams coconut flakes
100 grams cashews, raw
50 grams cranberries, dried
1 tbsp coconut oil
1 tsp maple syrup

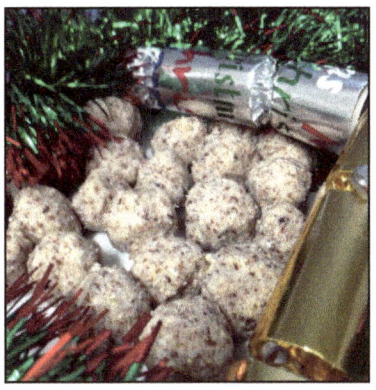

Procedure

1. Blend all ingredients in a high-powered blender or food processor until mixture crumbles and comes away from the sides of the blender/processor.
2. Remove mixture and shape into balls.
3. Refrigerate for at least 30 minutes before serving.

Servings: 15

Yield: 15 balls

Total Time: 40 minutes

Nutrition Facts

Nutrition (per serving): 95 calories, 7.6g total fat, 0mg cholesterol, 3.4mg sodium, 82.5mg potassium, 6.3g carbohydrates, 1.5g fibre, 1.2g sugar, 1.7g protein.

DF, GF, V, VG

The proanthocyanidins in cranberries can help urinary tract infections by acting as a barrier to bacteria. They may also assist in lowering bacteria in other areas of the body (www.whfoods.com).

Curried Cauliflower Bites

1/2 medium cauliflower, cut into florets
1 tbsp olive oil
1 tbsp lemon juice
1 tbsp curry powder
1/2 tsp coriander seed, ground
1/4 tsp cumin seeds, ground
1/4 tsp turmeric, ground
1/4 tsp cayenne pepper
1/2 tsp sumac

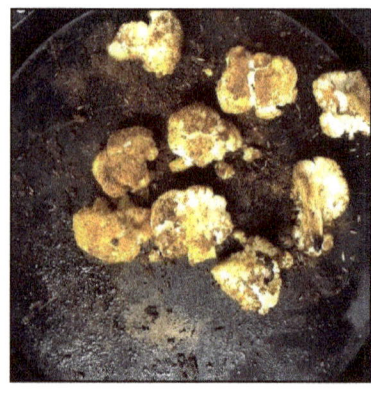

Procedure

1. Preheat the oven to 190 degrees C.
2. Place the cauliflower florets on a tray.
3. Mix the oil and lemon juice together and drizzle over the florets; toss lightly with your hands.
4. Mix the dried spices together in a bowl.
5. Transfer the cauliflower florets to the bowl or plastic bag and toss to coat evenly with the spice mix.
6. Arrange the florets on the tray and place in the preheated oven.
7. Cook for 15 - 20 minutes, then turn the florets with tongs, and return to the oven for another 15 minutes or until lightly browned.
8. Serve with yoghurt or a tahini/lemon dressing.

Servings: 2

Total Time: 35 minutes

Nutrition Facts

Nutrition (per serving): 115 calories, 7.9g total fat, 0mg cholesterol, 88.7mg sodium, 517.9mg potassium, 10.8g carbohydrates, 4.3g fibre, 3.1g sugar, 3.4g protein.

Dukkah

100 grams sesame seeds

60 grams hazelnuts and pistachios

1 tbsp cumin seeds

1 tsp caraway seed

1 tsp dried thyme

2 tbsp coriander seeds

1/2 tsp Himalayan salt

1/2 tsp peppercorns

1 tsp mint, dried

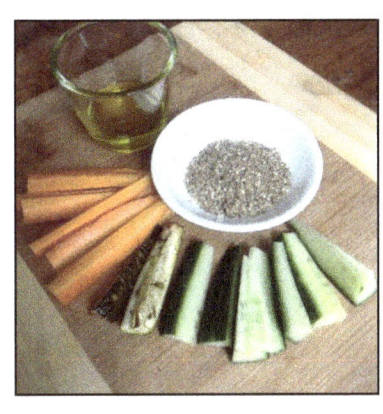

Procedure

1. Dry toast all ingredients in a non-stick pan over medium heat, stirring constantly to avoid burning.
2. Allow to cool.
3. Pulse in a food processor to a coarse blend.
4. Store in an air-tight jar.

Servings: 10

Total Time: 10 minutes

Nutrition Facts

Nutrition (per serving): 112 calories, 9.6g total fat, 0mg cholesterol, 122mg sodium, 165.8mg potassium, 6g carbohydrates, 3.3g fibre, <1g sugar, 3.4g protein.

DF, GF, V, VG

Dukkah is an Egyptian mixture of roasted nuts, seeds and spices. It can be used as a seasoning in cooking or served with fingers of whole meal sourdough.

Recipe Tips

Serve with olive oil and vegetable sticks; e.g. carrot, zucchini, cucumber.

Flax Crackers

1/2 cup flax seeds, ground

1 whole egg

1 tsp chia seeds

1 tsp poppy seeds

1 tsp dried rosemary (or other dried herbs), crushed

1 pinch Himalayan salt

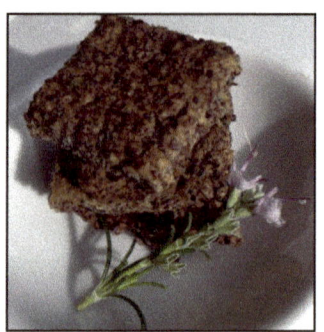

Procedure

1. Preheat oven to 180 degrees Celsius.
2. Mix all ingredients well with a fork.
3. Let mixture sit for 5 minutes to absorb some of the water, and make a thick paste.
4. Spread over baking paper with back of a dessert spoon, to 1mm thick.
5. Use a long knife to score 18 squares (3 columns, 6 rows).
6. Bake in preheated oven for 10 minutes, then remove and flip crackers over.
7. Bake for a further 5 minutes, remove and cool. Store in an airtight jar.

Servings: 4

Yield: 18 crackers

Total Time: 20 minutes

Nutrition Facts

Nutrition (per serving): 128 calories, 9.9g total fat, 46.5mg cholesterol, 96.7mg sodium, 184.7mg potassium, 6.3g carbohydrates, 5.7g fibre, <1g sugar, 5.3g protein.

DF, FOD, GF, V, VG

Recipe Tips

These are a rough-textured, fibrous cracker.

Adding 1/2 cup grated parmesan to the mix creates a more workable 'dough' that can be rolled out more easily. The same instructions apply.

Delicious with Cauliflower Hummus or Roast Capsicum dip.

Fruit Jellies

2 oranges, juiced
1 lime, juiced
1 pinch stevia (or to taste)
10 grams gelatin
2 tbsp boiling water

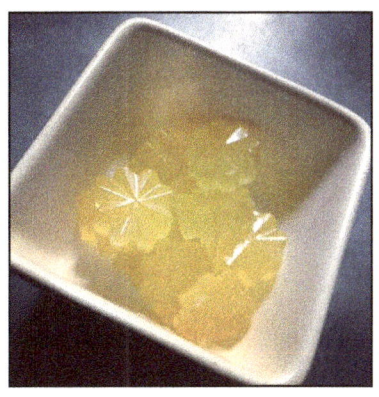

Procedure

1. Combine orange and lime juice. Add stevia to taste.
2. Combine gelatin with boiling water and stir quickly to dissolve gelatin.
3. Pour gelatin mix into juice and stir well.
4. Pour mixture into silicone moulds or an ice cube tray.
5. Refrigerate at least 30 minutes.
6. Store in the refrigerator in an airtight jar.

Servings: 5

Yield: 10 pieces

Total Time: 35 minutes

Nutrition Facts

Nutrition (per serving): 46 calories, <1g total fat, 0mg cholesterol, 9.8mg sodium, 147.1mg potassium, 11.9g carbohydrates, 2.1g fibre, 8.8g sugar, <1g protein.

DF, FOD, GF

Citrus fruits have powerful antibiotic and antioxidant effects. These jellies are a delicious alternative to commercial lollies. Check and adjust sweetness before cooling.

Not Toblerone

100 grams almonds
50 grams macadamia
30 grams coconut oil
1 tsp stevia
0.5 tsp vanilla extract
10 grams 85% cocoa chocolate (e.g. Lindt)

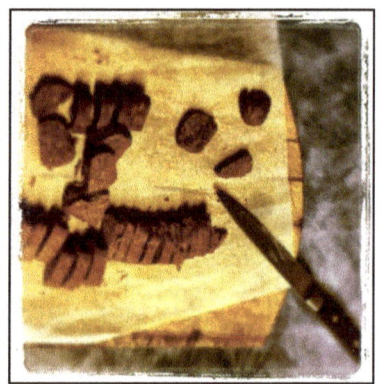

Procedure

1. Process all ingredients in your Thermomix or food processor until you have a wet dough consistency.
2. Put the mixture onto baking paper and shape into a long sausage, about 2 - 3cm thick. Rolling carefully like a sushi roll works well.
3. Wrap the sausage in baking paper, place on a tray and freeze for at least one hour.
4. Remove the sausage from the freezer, unwrap and cut into ten pieces (ten serves).
5. Keeps well in the freezer or refrigerator. Enjoy!

Servings: 10

Total Time: 1 hour and 15 minutes

Nutrition Facts

Nutrition (per serving): 126 calories, 12.2g total fat, <1mg cholesterol, <1mg sodium, 96.4mg potassium, 3.3g carbohydrates, 1.8g fibre, <1g sugar, 2.6g protein.

GF, V

Power Bites

1/4 cup sunflower seeds
1/4 cup pumpkin seeds
1/4 cup shredded coconut
2 tbsp flax seeds, ground
1 tbsp chia seeds
2 tbsp tahini
1 tsp vanilla extract
1 tbsp strawberry jam, 100% fruit (e.g. St Dalfour)

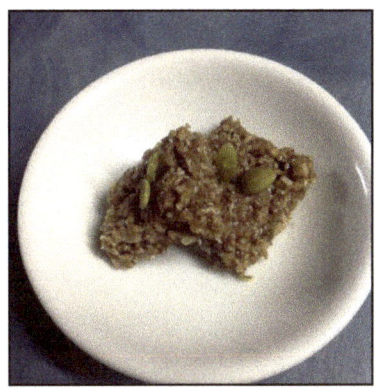

Procedure

1. Blend seeds and coconut in a food processor until crumbly.
2. Add remaining ingredients and pulse to combine.
3. Pour into a small dish lined with baking paper and press firmly.
4. Refrigerate 15 minutes.
5. Cut into 20 squares and store in refrigerator.

Servings: 20

Yield: 20 pieces

Total Time: 20 minutes

Nutrition Facts

Nutrition (per serving): 32 calories, 2.2g total fat, 0mg cholesterol, 25mg sodium, 42.1mg potassium, 2.5g carbohydrates, 1.1g fibre, <1g sugar, <1g protein.

DF, GF, V, VG

A tasty power-house snack that's a good source of healthy fats and fibre.

Scrumptious Mushroom Walnut Pate

1 onion chopped
3 sprigs thyme
1 clove garlic, minced
1 tbsp olive oil
500 grams mushrooms (any)
1 cup toasted walnuts
1 tsp miso paste
1/2 tsp lemon rind, finely grated
1 tsp cracked black pepper
1 cup vegetable stock
3 tsp gelatin powder (or agar)

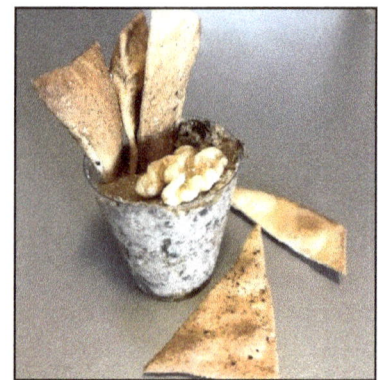

Procedure

1. Heat a frypan over medium; lightly toast the walnuts - set aside.
2. Sautee the onion, thyme, garlic and olive oil over medium heat.
3. Add mushrooms and cook 8 - 10 minutes, turning to brown.
4. Transfer the pan ingredients to a Thermomix or food processor.
5. Blend walnuts, miso, pepper and lemon rind in a food processor.
6. Blend until the desired consistency is reached - lightly crumbly, or well-blended. In a Thermomix, try 15 seconds, Sp 5.
7. Use a spatula to transfer the pate to individual shot glasses, or a glass container, then refrigerate 15 minutes.
8. Heat the stock in a glass jug or milk saucepan (for pouring) and add the gelatin or agar agar powder; stir well to dissolve.
9. Pour the stock gently into a teaspoon held just over the surface of the pate – to avoid the mix going cloudy.
10. Refrigerate for 30 minutes before serving. Top with fresh herbs if desired; serve with lavash or vegetable sticks.

Servings: 10

Yield: 10 serves (roughly 10 x 30g shot glasses)

Total Time: 1 hour and 20 minutes

Nutrition Facts

Nutrition (per serving): 137 calories, 9.7g total fat, 0mg cholesterol, 1355.2mg sodium, 319.6mg potassium, 11g carbohydrates, 2.1g fibre, 6.9g sugar, 4.4g protein.

Source

Source: Adapted from www.scalingbackblog.com

Strawberry Roses

6 medium strawberries

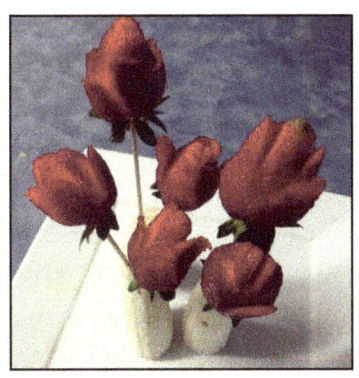

Procedure

1. Wash strawberries well.
2. Using a small knife, hold the base of one strawberry with your thumb and slice downwards (carefully); push open slightly to make a petal.
3. Turn the strawberry around and slice another three petals using the same method.
4. Moving up slightly toward the tip of the strawberry, slice another two or three petals in the gap between the bottom petals, pushing them open slightly as you go.
5. At the tip of the strawberry, slice downwards and push the split open.
6. Gently insert a skewer into the base of the strawberry (through the green leaves), but not all the way through.
7. Can be served in a vase, or with the skewers anchored in other fruits (e.g. banana).

Servings: 2

Total Time: 10 minutes

Nutrition Facts

Nutrition (per serving): 12 calories, <1g total fat, 0mg cholesterol, <1mg sodium, 55.1mg potassium, 2.8g carbohydrates, <1g fibre, 1.8g sugar, <1g protein.

DF, FOD, GF, V, VG

Strawberries perish rapidly - purchase and use on the day of preparation. Strawberries are often treated with fungicides, so purchase organic strawberries where possible.

Zucchini Avocado Hummus

1 avocado
3 zucchinis, coarsely chopped
1 garlic clove
2 tbsp tahini
2 tbsp lemon juice
1 pinch cumin seeds, ground
1 tbsp olive oil
1/2 tsp sumac (optional)

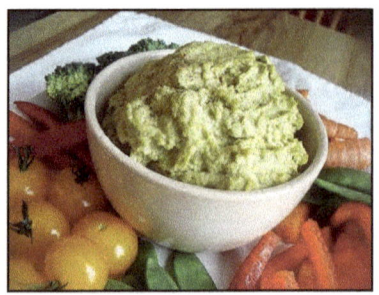

Procedure

1. Puree all ingredients except oil and sumac.
2. Transfer hummus to a serving dish and smear the top flat with a spoon.
3. Drizzle oil over the top and sprinkle with sumac (or paprika if preferred).
4. Serve with carrot sticks, snow peas, green beans and capsicum sticks.

Servings: 16

Total Time: 5 minutes

Nutrition Facts

Nutrition (per serving): 46 calories, 3.8g total fat, 0mg cholesterol, 10.9mg sodium, 174.7mg potassium, 3.1g carbohydrates, 1.4g fibre, 1.1g sugar, 1.1g protein.

DF, GF, V, VG

Zucchinis are a low-GI vegetable that has antioxidant, blood sugar, anti-cancer, anti-inflammatory and antimicrobial benefits. It is an excellent source of copper and manganese (www.whfoods.com).

Recipe Tips

This mixture won't keep well –use within 2 hours of preparation and ensure the olive oil covers the surface of the prepared dip, to reduce browning.

8 Desserts

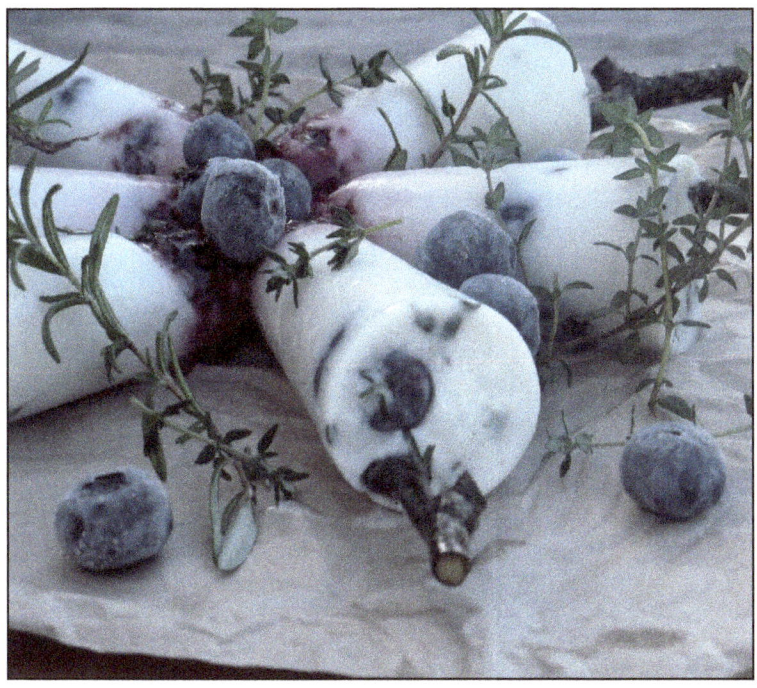

Blood Orange Jelly

2 blood oranges, juice only
10 grams gelatin
100 ml water, boiling
1 serve blueberry sorbet

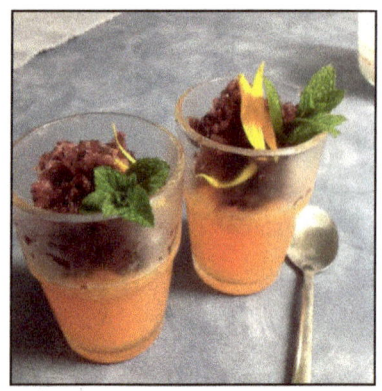

Procedure

1. Juice blood oranges into a bowl.
2. Pour boiling water into a glass.
3. Add gelatin to the boiling water and stir until gelatin dissolves.
4. Pour gelatin mixture into orange juice and stir well.
5. Pour orange juice into two desert cups and refrigerate until set.
6. Serve with blueberry sorbet if desired.
7. Add whipped coconut cream if desired.

Servings: 2

Total Time: 40 minutes

Nutrition Facts

Nutrition (per serving): 116 calories, <1g total fat, 0mg cholesterol, 25.1mg sodium, 350.4mg potassium, 28.8g carbohydrates, 4.8g fibre, 6g sugar, 2.3g protein.

DF, FOD, GF

Blueberry Sorbet

65 grams blueberries, frozen
4 ice cubes
1 tbsp lemon or lime juice
1 pinch stevia (optional)

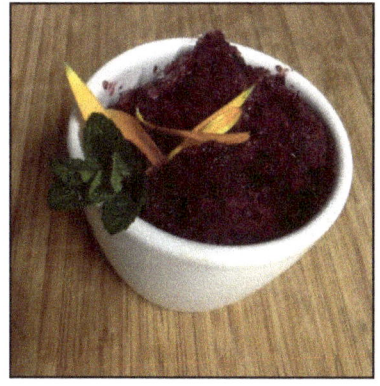

Procedure

1. Blend all ingredients in a food processor until finely crushed.
2. Serve immediately.

Servings: 2

Total Time: 5 minutes

Nutrition Facts

Nutrition (per serving): 20 calories, <1g total fat, 0mg cholesterol, <1mg sodium, 33mg potassium, 5.2g carbohydrates, <1g fibre, 3.4g sugar, <1g protein.

DF, FOD, GF, V, VG

Coconut Ice Cream

2 cans coconut milk, organic (or one milk, one cream)

2 tsp arrowroot

1/2 cup maple syrup

1 tsp vanilla extract

1/2 tsp stevia (optional)

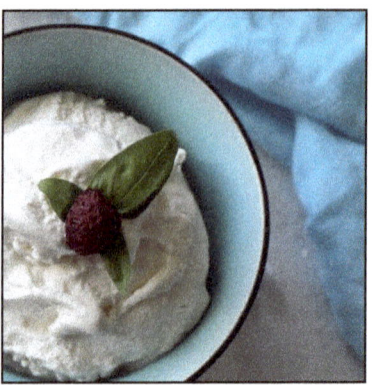

Procedure

1. Pour the coconut milk (and cream, if using) into a saucepan over low heat and gently heat through.
2. Mix a little warmed milk with arrowroot; stir to remove lumps.
3. Add arrowroot mix to the saucepan and stir continuously over low heat for 10 minutes, until the mixture thickens into a custard.
4. Add the maple syrup and vanilla; stir to combine and cook another 2 - 3 minutes. Add stevia to taste, if desired.
5. Remove from the heat and put the base of the saucepan into a cold-water bath (a sink filled with icy water will do).
6. Stir until the mixture cools, blend/ food process.
7. Freeze for 30 minutes, then remove and blend again.
8. Repeat the freeze/blend step another two times, then return to the freezer and freeze until set.
9. This ice cream needs to be softened for 5 - 10 minutes before scooping. Fruit can also be added to the mixture during setting.

Servings: 10

Total Time: 4 hours and 35 minutes

Nutrition Facts

Nutrition (per serving): 133 calories, 9.7g total fat, 0mg cholesterol, 7.8mg sodium, 133.5mg potassium, 12.4g carbohydrates, <1g fibre, 10.8g sugar, <1g protein.

DF, GF, V, VG

Fruit Icy Poles

3/4 cup blueberries
1/2 cup coconut milk
1 cup coconut water
1/2 tsp vanilla extract

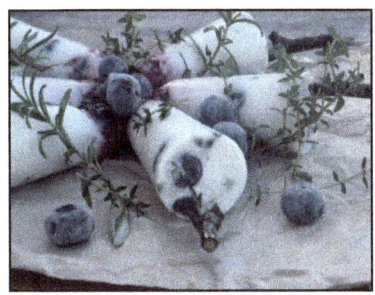

Procedure

1. Mix vanilla extract, coconut milk and coconut water together.
2. Distribute the mixture evenly between four icy pole moulds.
3. Distribute blueberries between the four icy pole moulds.
4. Insert the sticks and freeze for at least four hours.

Servings: 4

Yield: Four icy poles.

Total Time: 4 hours and 5 minutes

Nutrition Facts

Nutrition (per serving): 89 calories, 6.5g total fat, 0mg cholesterol, 66.9mg sodium, 241.3mg potassium, 7.9g carbohydrates, 1.3g fibre, 4.3g sugar, 1.1g protein.

DF, FOD, GF, V, VG

Source

Source: Melanie White

Image supplied by Belinda McDonald of The Green Kitchen.

www.thegreenkitchen.co.nz

Grasshopper Mint Slice

1 whole avocado, Hass
4 tbsp coconut oil
1 cup shredded coconut
1/2 tsp peppermint extract
4 tbsp coconut oil
1/2 tsp stevia
4 tbsp cacao powder (rounded spoons)
1/2 tsp vanilla extract
1 pinch Himalayan salt

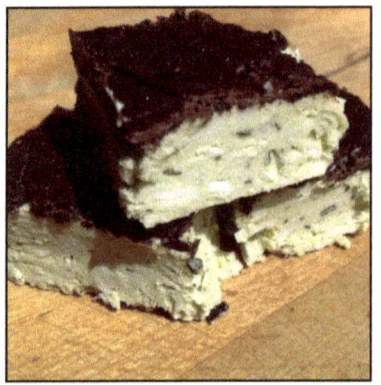

Procedure

1. Line a square baking dish with baking paper.
2. Place the avocado, coconut oil, shredded coconut, peppermint extract in a blender or food processor and blend until smooth with some flecks of coconut remaining.
3. Smooth into the pan and place in the freezer for 10 minutes.
4. Meanwhile, melt the coconut oil in a saucepan until liquid. Remove from the heat and add stevia (optional), cacao powder, vanilla extract and salt.
5. Pour chocolate mix over the avocado layer and return to the freezer.
6. After 10 minutes, remove from the freezer and cut into 10 squares.

Servings: 10

Yield: 10 pieces

Total Time: 30 minutes

Nutrition Facts

Nutrition (per serving): 197 calories, 20.5g total fat, 0mg cholesterol, 34.6mg sodium, 153.6mg potassium, 4.4g carbohydrates, 3.5g fibre, <1g sugar, 1.5g protein.

DF, GF, V, VG

Source

Source: Melanie White

Mini Pavlovas

4 egg whites
1/2 tsp stevia
2 tbsp raspberries
8 large strawberries, chopped
1 tbsp water
1 pinch stevia

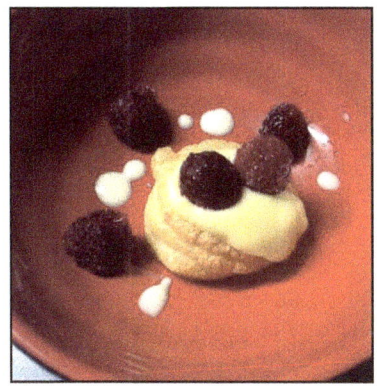

Procedure

1. Preheat the oven to 120 degrees Celsius.
2. Beat egg whites until fluffy.
3. Add stevia and beat until stiff peaks form.
4. Spoon or pipe meringue mix onto a tray lined with baking paper.
5. Bake until dry to touch (about 1 hour), then leave in the oven with door ajar to cool completely.
6. Add strawberries to a saucepan with water and stevia to taste.
7. Simmer strawberries and mash well.
8. To assemble, Place meringues on a plate and add raspberries.
9. Top with strawberry sauce, or alternatively, with some stevia-sweetened Greek yoghurt.

Servings: 2

Total Time: 1 hour and 15 minutes

Nutrition Facts

Nutrition (per serving): 62 calories, <1g total fat, 0mg cholesterol, 111.9mg sodium, 230.7mg potassium, 6.9g carbohydrates, 1.9g fibre, 4.3g sugar, 7.9g protein.

DF, FOD, GF, V

Source

Source: Recipe provided by Sam Ricza, Mossy Point. NSW

Orange Coconut Sorbet

1 whole blood orange or other orange, cut into segments.

4 tbsp coconut milk

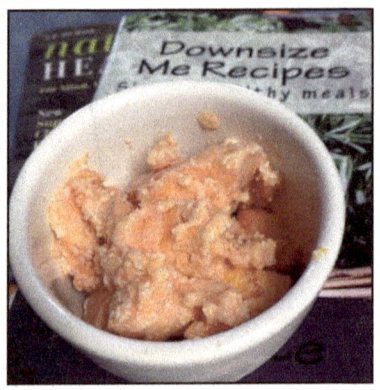

Procedure

1. Pour the coconut milk into an ice cube tray and freeze.
2. Put the orange segments into a container and freeze (min. 4 hours).
3. When properly frozen, blend the orange and coconut milk.
4. Serve immediately.

Servings: 1

Total Time: 4 hours and 5 minutes

Nutrition Facts

Nutrition (per serving): 125 calories, 4g total fat, 0mg cholesterol, 0mg sodium, 333mg potassium, 22.5g carbohydrates, 4.4g fibre, <1g sugar, 2.2g protein.

DF, FOD, GF, V, VG

Recipe Tips

Add stevia to taste.

Raw Boysenberry Cheesecake

1/3 cup almonds
1/3 cup pecans
1/3 cup sunflower seeds
1 tsp vanilla extract
1 tbsp coconut oil
1 cup cashews, soaked
1 tsp vanilla extract
1 tsp maple syrup or honey
1 tsp lemon juice
1 cup boysenberries

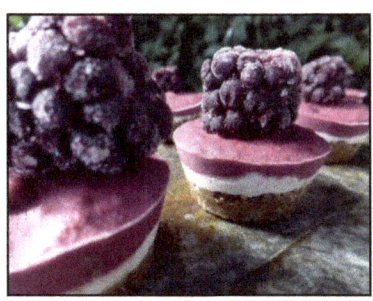

Procedure

1. Soak cashews overnight, then drain before use.
2. Puree the almonds, pecans, sunflower seeds & vanilla extract.
3. Add coconut oil and pulse to combine.
4. Press mix into the bottoms of individual muffin pans and refrigerate.
5. Puree cashews in a food processor until smooth and creamy.
6. Add vanilla, lemon juice, 1 tsp vanilla extract and maple syrup.
7. Divide the mixture in two; pour half into the muffin pans; refrigerate.
8. Blend the remaining cashew mixture with 1/2 cup of the berries.
9. Pour berry layer over first layer (when set) and refrigerate.
10. Allow 60 mins before serving. Top with remaining berries.

Servings: 8

Yield: 8 cheesecakes

Total Time: 1 hour and 20 minutes

Nutrition Facts

Nutrition (per serving): 113 calories, 9g total fat, 0mg cholesterol, 3.3mg sodium, 126.9mg potassium, 7g carbohydrates, 2.3g fibre, 2.4g sugar, 2.4g protein.

DF, GF, V, VG

Source

Recipe & image supplied by Belinda McDonald
www.thegreenkitchen.co.nz

Strawberry Cheesecakes

300 grams Greek Yoghurt
200 grams Ricotta cheese
1 cup strawberries
1 tbsp maple syrup
1 tsp vanilla extract
1 sachet gelatin
100 mL boiling water
1/2 cup almonds (base)
1/2 cup pecans (base)
1/2 cup cashews (base)
1 tsp coconut oil (base)
1 tsp vanilla extract (base)

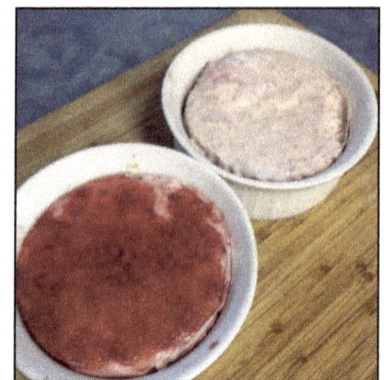

Procedure

1. Preheat the oven to 180 degrees C.
2. Blend base ingredients in a food processor until a thick mixture forms.
3. Line four small ramekins with baking paper; distribute the nut mix evenly between them, and press into the base; bake 10 minutes.
4. Mix yoghurt, ricotta and maple syrup and vanilla well, until evenly mixed (blend if desired).
5. Dissolve the gelatin in boiling water and stir through the yoghurt.
6. Puree half the strawberries and stir through the yoghurt mix, then slice and add the remaining strawberries; mix well.
7. Refrigerate until set (about 2 hours).

Servings: 4

Total Time: 2 hours and 30 minutes

Nutrition Facts

Nutrition (per serving): 553 calories, 35.1g total fat, 15.5mg cholesterol, 199.6mg sodium, 440.7mg potassium, 45.4g carbohydrates, 4.3g fibre, 31.5g sugar, 19.4g protein.

GF, V

Recipe Tips

Reserve a little strawberry puree and add 1 tsp of dissolved gelatin, then top the set cheesecake with this and refrigerate.

9 Basics

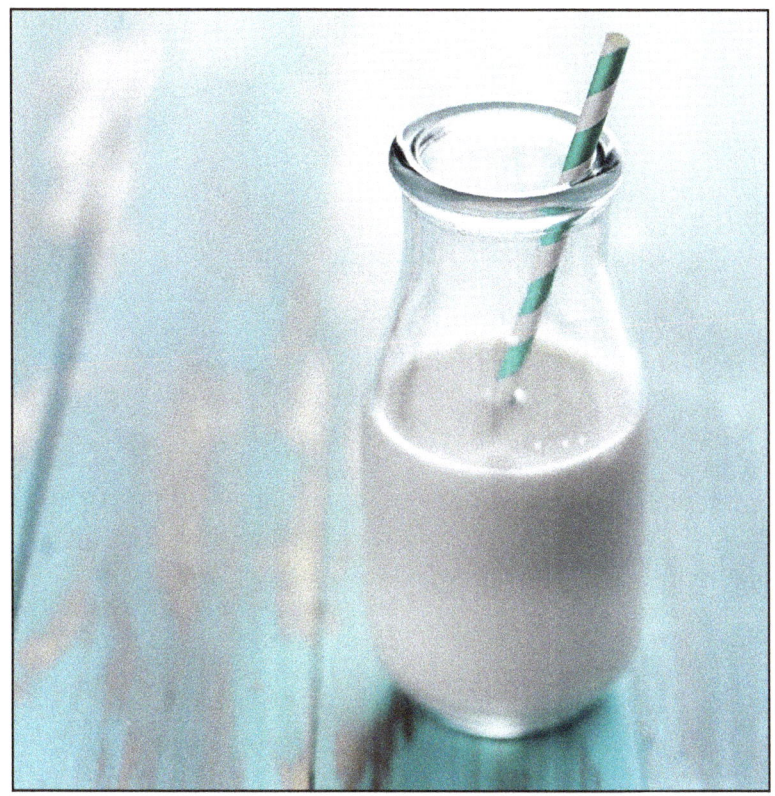

Almond Milk

1 cup almonds, whole
2 cups water
1/2 tsp vanilla extract
1 pinch Himalayan salt

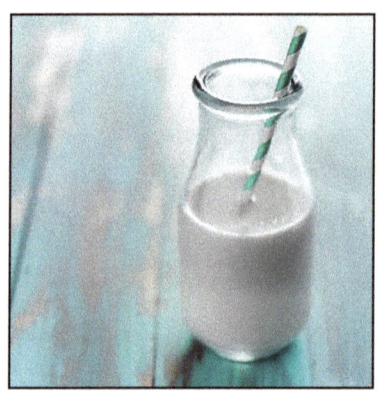

Procedure

1. Cover almonds with water and soak for at least 4 hours, or overnight.
2. Discard soak water and rinse almonds.
3. Puree almonds, 2 cups fresh water, vanilla and salt in a food processor until smooth (about 2 minutes on high).
4. Pour the mixture through a cheesecloth or fine-mesh cloth into a bowl.
5. Hold the cloth around the remaining pulp, and start twisting the cloth above the pulp, to remove moisture.
6. Transfer the pulp to a separate container for later use.
7. Transfer the strained almond milk to a bottle that seals well.
8. Store in the refrigerator and use within 5 days.

Servings: 4

Total Time: 4 hours and 10 minutes

Nutrition Facts

Nutrition (per serving): 325 calories, 9.5g total fat, 13.5g carbohydrates, 13.5g sugar, 3g protein.

DF, FOD, GF, V, VG

This drink is a good source of vitamin E, vitamin D and calcium.

Beef bone broth

1 joint roasted beef, bones and cartilage attached
4 stalks celery, chopped
1 carrot
1 bay leaf
1 onion, finely diced
2 tbsp apple cider vinegar
1 pinch Himalayan salt
5 cups water

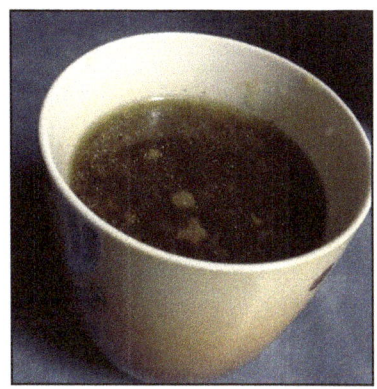

Procedure

1. Place leftover roast beef bone (or raw bone) in a slow cooker.
2. Add remaining ingredients and simmer for 24 - 48 hours.
3. Skim fat from the top; strain stock; remove then discard bones.
4. Serve as a soup or freeze in batches for soup stock. Keeps in the refrigerator for up to two weeks.

Servings: 4

Total Time: 24 hours and 10 minutes

Nutrition Facts

Nutrition (per serving): 58 calories, 1.9g total fat, 8mg cholesterol, 65.4mg sodium, 235.3mg potassium, 6.2g carbohydrates, 1.8g fibre, 3.1g sugar, 3.6g protein.

DF, GF

Good immunity starts in the gut. The gelatin in bone broth is an excellent gut-healer that has been used since ancient times. Apart from supporting digestion, bone broth is an excellent source of easily-absorbed minerals (www.westonaprice.org).

Recipe Tips

Use fish, chicken, beef or other bones to make different-flavoured broths. Fish and chicken bones cook for ~24 hours, and other bones can be roasted up to 72 hours to extract flavour. Can be used for reductions.

Cauliflower Pizza or Tortilla Wrap

2 cups cauliflower, grated

2 small eggs, lightly beaten

1 tsp rosemary (or other herbs), fresh, finely chopped

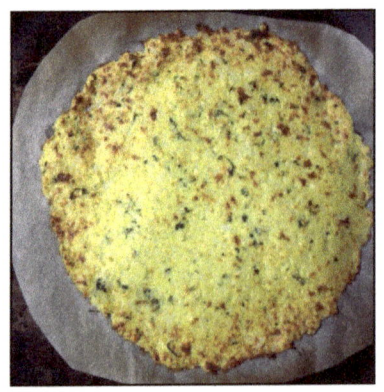

Procedure

1. Preheat the oven to 180 degrees Celsius.
2. Put grated cauliflower in a non-stick pan or glass microwave dish and cook for 5 mins. Cool, then squeeze until almost dry in a paper towel.
3. Whip through the egg (or egg white) and fresh herbs.
4. Line a large tray with baking paper.
5. Pour two mounds of cauliflower mix on the tray and smooth into circles, about 20 - 25cm diameter.
6. Bake for 15 minutes in the oven or until golden, then turn over.
7. Bake again for 10- 15 minutes until golden.
8. Use as a soft tortilla or add pizza toppings and bake.

Servings: 1

Yield: 2 bases/tortillas

Total Time: 35 minutes

Nutrition Facts

Nutrition (per serving): 194 calories, 10.1g total fat, 372mg cholesterol, 202.2mg sodium, 740.7mg potassium, 10.8g carbohydrates, 4.1g fibre, 4.2g sugar, 16.4g protein.

DF, GF, V

Recipe Tips

These will stay fairly firm but flexible.

Preserved Lemon

4 whole lemons, cut into sixths

4 tbsp lemon juice, freshly squeezed

2 tbsp Himalayan salt

1 sprig dill (fresh herb) (optional)

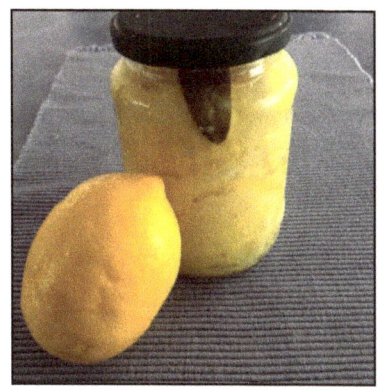

Procedure

1. Put cut lemons into a sterilized jar, sprinkling salt on each layer.
2. Press lemons down firmly.
3. Pour lemon juice over the top.
4. Seal the jar well and store for 3 - 4 weeks in the refrigerator before use.

Servings: 24

Yield: 24 pieces

Preparation Time: 10 minutes

Nutrition Facts

Nutrition (per serving): 4 calories, <1g total fat, 0mg cholesterol, 582mg sodium, 29.2mg potassium, 2.1g carbohydrates, <1g fibre, <1g sugar, <1g protein.

DF, FOD, GF, V, VG

Wash and scrub lemons well before use to ensure any protective wax or other treatment is removed before use. Even better – grow your own.

Sauerkraut

1 whole cabbage (red, green or white), shredded
1 cup kale, finely chopped
1 tsp caraway seeds
1 tsp juniper berries
1 bay leaf
2 tsp Himalayan salt
2 tbsp liquid whey (from strained yoghurt or kefir)

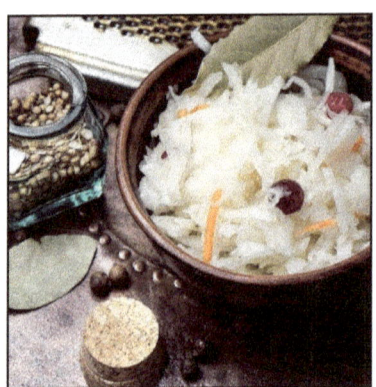

Procedure

1. Sterilize jar and all implements in boiling water before use.
2. Put shredded cabbage and kale into a bowl with the salt.
3. Use a kraut pounder or meat mallet to gently pound the cabbage, mixing while pounding (or massage with your hands) for 5 - 10 mins.
4. Mix through caraway seeds, juniper berries and bay leaf (crumbled).
5. Pack tightly into a mason jar, or other jar with a tight seal, and push down firmly so the liquid rises above the cabbage.
6. Seal jar, leave on a bench, regularly packing down over 24 hours.
7. If liquid has not risen over the cabbage after 24 hours, dissolve 1 tsp salt in 1 cup water; add enough to fully submerge cabbage.
8. Seal the jar, ferment (away from sunlight) for 7 days then refrigerate.

Servings: 6

Total Time: 3 weeks

Nutrition Facts

Nutrition (per serving): 12 calories, <1g total fat, <1mg cholesterol, 62mg sodium, 95.7mg potassium, 2.3g carbohydrates, <1g fibre, <1g sugar, <1g protein.

DF, FOD, GF, V, VG * People on a low FODMAP diet may or may not tolerate sauerkraut.

Whipped Coconut Cream

100 ml coconut milk

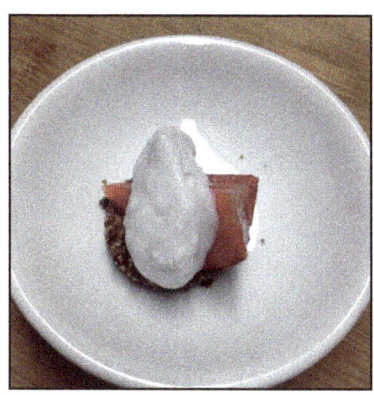

Procedure

1. Refrigerate coconut milk overnight.
2. Skim solids from the top (cream) and place into a bowl.
3. Whip with an electric beater (or with food processor) for 3 - 5 minutes.
4. Serve 1 tbsp with your favourite dessert.

Servings: 2

Total Time: 5 minutes

Nutrition Facts

Nutrition (per serving): 99 calories, 10.7g total fat, 0mg cholesterol, 6.5mg sodium, 110mg potassium, 1.4g carbohydrates, 1g protein.

DF, FOD, GF, V, VG

Index

A
AK-47 2
Almond Milk 102
Asian Salad with Salmon . 30
Asparagus with Lemon and Almonds 55

B
Bahmi Goreng 31
Baked Egg with Pesto Mushroom 10
Beef bone broth 103
Beef Meatballs in Tomato Mushroom Sauce (Red Rose Cafe) 32
Beetslaw 56
Blood Orange Jelly 92
Blueberry Sorbet 93
Breakfast Mug Cake 11
Breakfast Tapas 12

C
Capsi Egg 13
Carrot and Cauliflower Soup 23
Carrot and Fennel Soup ... 24
Carrot and Hazelnut Salad 57
Carrot and Kale Salad 58
Cauliflower Pizza or Tortilla Wrap 104
Celery Soup 25
Chai Tea Mix 3
Chef's Salad with Fruit 33
Chia Pudding 14
Chicken and Black Rice Lunchbox 34
Chicken Fritters (The Muffin Shop) 35
Chicken Kale Soup with Probiotic Saurkraut 26
Chicken Stir Fry 36

Chicken with Beetroot, Carrot, Apple and Ginger Salad 37
Chimichurri 73
Chimichurri Steak with Lemon Asparagus and Sweet Potato Chips 38
Christmas Balls 81
Coconut Ice Cream 94
Coleslaw 59
Cucumber and Fennel Salad 60
Curried Cauliflower Bites .. 82

D
Dukkah 83

E
Eggplant Parmagiana 61
Eggplant, Tomato and Fetta Salad (Grumpy and Sweetheart's) 62

F
Flax Crackers 84
Flaxible Smoothie 15
Fruit Icy Poles 95
Fruit Jellies 85
Fruity Chia Pudding 16

G
Golden Oatmeal Smoothie . 4
Grapefruit Breakfast Margarita 5
Grasshopper Mint Slice 96
Greek Salad 64
Gremolata 74

I
Indian Chicken 39
Indian Spinach 65
Indonesian Beef Stirfry 40

L
Life Saver Muesli 17

M
Mini Pavlovas 97

Mushroom Burgers 41
N
Nasi Goreng 42
Not Toblerone 86
O
Orange AC juice 6
Orange Coconut Sorbet 98
P
Pizza, low fat Chicken 43
Pizza, Supreme 44
Power Bites 87
Preserved Lemon 105
Preserved Lemon Dressing
.... 75
R
Raspberry Jam 76
Raspberry Macarina
(Rivermouth Cafe) 7
Raw Boysenberry
Cheesecake 99
Revitaliser (Moruya Health
Cafe) 8
Ridiculously Good Pancakes
.... 18
Roasted Sweet Potato and
Fig Salad with Balsamic
Glaze 66
Rocking Breakfast Smoothie
.... 19
S
Satisfying Chicken Salad .. 45
Sauerkraut 106
Scrumptious Mushroom
Walnut Pate 88

Shaved Fennel and Kale
Salad 67
Silverbeet Salad Wraps 46
Simple Avo and Pea Salad
.... 68
Soft Lamb Tortillas 47
Souper Soup 27
Spaghetti Squash
Bolognaise 48
Spicy Avocado Sauce 77
Spring Tuna Salad 49
Strawberry Cheesecakes 100
Strawberry Roses 89
Summer Stir Fry 50
Super Pesto 78
Surf and Turf with Spicy Avo
Sauce 51
Sweet Potato and Orange
Pancakes 20
Sweet Potato Chips 69
T
Tabbouleh 70
Tahini Lemon Dressing 79
Tasty Beef Burgers 52
Tuna Bolognaise 53
V
Vegan Sweet Potato
Pancakes 21
Vegetable Soup 28
W
Whipped Coconut Cream 107
Winter Greens Salad 71
Z
Zucchini Avocado Hummus
.... 90

www.ingramcontent.com/pod-product-compliance
Lightning Source LLC
Chambersburg PA
CBHW062102290426
44110CB00022B/2682